the Rec[i]
Living Without Disease

❖

Volume One
What's To Discuss? Let's Eat!

❖

Volume Two
The Recipe For Healthy Living
& Optimal Recipes!

❖

Volume Three
The Science Of Living Healthfully

❖

Volume Four
Health Or Disease?

❖

AAJONUS VONDERPLANITZ

Author of the life-changing book on living free of disease:
The Primal Diet; We Want To Live

Carnelian Bay Castle Press
Santa Monica

Published by
CARNELIAN BAY CASTLE PRESS, LLC
P.O. Box 66663
Los Angeles, CA 90066

Jacket design by Kari Lucille Jacob

Library of Congress Cataloging-in-publication Data

Vonderplanitz, Aajonus, 1947-

The recipe for living without disease / Aajonus Vonderplanitz.

p. cm.

Includes bibliographical references and index.

Contents: v. 1. What's to discuss? Let's eat! -- v. 2. The recipe for healthy living & optimal recipes! -- v. 3. The science of living healthfully -- v. 4. Health or disease?

ISBN 978-1-889356-84-6 (alk. Paper)

1. Raw food diet. I. Title.

RM237.5 .V665 2002

613.2'6—dc21   200203365

Printed in the Thomson Press India Ltd.
First Edition, 2002
Second Printing 2005
Third Printing 2007

CONTENTS

Volume Three

The Science Of Living Healthfully

Volume Four

Health Or Disease?

FOREWORD

All of my students reported that they learned as much from their sixteenth read of my book *The Primal Diet; We Want To Live, Vol. 1, Out Of The Grips Of Disease And Death (the story); and Vol. 2, Healthfully (the facts),*[1] as they did when they read it for the first time. The information in that book and this book is so contrary to the assumed medical perspective that I suggest everyone on the path to optimal health reread my books often for better clarity and understanding. Health awareness develops incrementally over time and with experience.

DEDICATION

To my son John Jeffrey Marshall,
Dennis Kruhm, Paul Kruhm, Lori Jacob, Lucille Jacob &
Family, James Stewart, James Hopson, Norman Fritz,
Pat Connolly, Greg Laur, and health-minded individuals.

DISCLAIMER

This material has been written and published solely for educational purposes. The reader understands that the author and publisher are not engaged in rendering medical advice or services. The author and publisher provide this information, and the reader accepts it, with the understanding that people act on it at their own risk. The author and publisher shall have neither liability or responsibility to any person or entity with respect to any loss, damage or injury caused, or alleged to be caused, directly or indirectly by the information contained in this book.

---

[1] Santa Monica, CA; Carnelian Bay Castle Press, 1997, 2005.

the Recipe for Living Without disease

———◇———

Volume One
What's To Discuss? Let's Eat!

—◇—

Volume Two
The Recipe For Healthy Living
& Optimal Recipes!

—◇—

Volume Three
The Science Of Living Healthfully

—◇—

Volume Four
Health Or Disease?

—◇—

Aajonus Vonderplanitz

Author of the life-changing book on living free of disease:
The Primal Diet; We Want To Live

We can live without fear of disease, disease-free.

Volume One

What's To Discuss? Let's Eat!

Chapter 1
Are We Safe?

According to the world-renowned Dr. Samuel Epstein, M.D., one of every 2.5 people develops cancer. Why has the cancer rate increased from 1 in 8,000 in the year 1906 to 1 in 2.5?

Considering all of the other diseases and those yet to come, what are our chances of developing disease in our lifetime? 100%?! What are the odds that hospitals, doctors, insurance companies and HMOs will decide that it is too expensive to treat us? How many insurance companies will deny us, or fail and seek bankruptcy? According to recent estimates, 50% of possible medical treatment is withheld because of cost-savings. Trends indicate that in 10 years, few people will have access to medical treatments other than drugs. Why do we continue to hear from the media that medical science is on the verge of freeing us from disease?

With the extremely low success-rate of medical treatments, what are the odds that medical therapies will be a waste of our time, money and health? What are the chances that we will get medical-induced diseases from doctors, hospitals and medication?

The Journal of American Medical Association reported from university research that conservatively, 137,000 hospital deaths and 2.1 million serious hospital injuries occur each year from medication. Additionally, consider the conservative estimate that the non-hospital-medication deaths and injuries may be 5 million per year. Plus, medical therapies cause over 2 million diseases per year. With those statistics, should we trust medical treatments? Do we want to risk those frightful odds?

Would we be more secure in living life-styles that insure better health and freedom from disease at a fraction of the cost of medical treatments?

How I Discovered What Health Is

I am compelled to tell my story. It may save many lives from falling into the same fate that I did with medical treatment. I am one of the statistics cited above. My experiences were traumatic and true. Often, they elicit emotionality, even hostility toward the medical system. However, I no longer live in anger or hostility. My life is wonderful now. I took responsibility and made it rich in health.

I was frequently sick after birth. I was administered pound after pound of medication without dietary change. Family, teachers, the media, doctors and scientists convinced me to believe that disease is a natural phenomenon to which mainly weak-minded individuals succumb. I was considered weak and useless. Instead of getting healthier with medical therapy, I got worse. Some people said that I suffered at the mercy of God, Karma or Nature. Others said that I was the product of genetic mishap.

I was conditioned to believe that a few pills or injections would cure my problems. Then I was led to believe that several pounds of pills or injections were needed. I was indoctrinated to believe that medication is all-important and that the quality of our food is of little consequence.

My first 20 years were full of illness including developmental autism. At 20, I was diagnosed with a stomach ulcer. Medical treatment turned the ulcer into cancer. The doctors treated me as if I were stupid if I did not do what they demanded. They told me that I would suffer "beyond belief" and die quickly. They traumatized me into believing that I had to let them cut and restructure my stomach, expose me to radiation and infuse me with chemotherapy.

Doctors did not tell me that for every one cancer cell that is burned by radiation a hundred million healthy cells are burned. I was not informed that radiation prevented billions of healthy cells from reproducing. They did not mention that radiation therapy would cause blood and bone cancers, cauterize my spine and greatly restrict movement. They did not inform me that for every one cancer cell poisoned by chemotherapy one billion healthy cells were poisoned. There was no mention that chemotherapy congested the lymph system and would cause me lymphoma. They did not tell me that all of their cancer treatments prevented proper healing, or that they would give me psoriasis and bursitis. They did not warn me that chemotherapy would damage my kidneys and bladder. I learned the hard way that, probably, I would not be able to live without a diaper.

The horror stories I heard, about what would happen if I did not attack the cancer, would have been a lot less traumatic than what I experienced with treatment. Doctors said that those therapies would be helpful and extend my life; possibly conquer my cancers. My life deteriorated rapidly within weeks after each therapy ended. The treatments rendered me suicidal in despair.

Rather than speak rationally about the facts of cancer-treatment, doctors terrorized me into believing them. I call it terrorism because their advice and stories left me so completely traumatized that I did anything they prescribe whether rational or not, based on true science or not.

Too late, I comprehended that the foundation and structure of medicine is disease not wellness. I learned that doctors know little or nothing about health and healing. I discovered that medical doctors' prejudices and fears do not accept rationale or empirical evidence when it comes to food, bacteria, virus, parasites, disease and pollution.

Doctors have been trained to attack microbes. We are treated with drugs that most often do not work. When they work, the effects are usually temporary and addictive. All drugs have side effects. After doctors crippled me and gave me a "definite" 3-months death-sentence, I began to reject medical therapies.

Through searching and trial and error, I discovered alternative approaches to wellness. One of my first realizations came a year after one of my doctors severed all of the vagus nerves to my stomach as treatment for the cancerous stomach ulcer. After the fact, he explained that I would never be able to eat fresh <u>raw</u> food again because my stomach would never again produce hydrochloric acid. After surgery, I noticed that foods did affect me radically. Consequently, I realized that food affects health.

When I was given the ultimate death-sentence a year after stomach surgery and suffering with a normal cooked diet, I experimented and ate the opposite of what the doctors prescribed. I discovered that I digested fresh raw foods very well, except for whole vegetables. I felt a little better.

Chapter 2
Origin of Disease

I began to explore theories that were not embraced by the medical profession. One theory with substantial supportive documentation is that we are industrially, environmentally, dietarily and medicinally poisoning ourselves into disease. That theory generated the movements toward ecology and healthfood. Very little contemporary scientific research has been funded to discover the truths proposed by those movements.

We have plenty of evidence that environmental pollution is hazardous and creates volatile toxins. We have proof that cooking and processing alter the chemical properties of food, destroying nutrients and creating volatile toxins. We know that deficiencies and volatile toxins cause disease. We simply need to connect the dots: <u>Deficiencies and toxicity</u>, not microbes, cause loss of cellular integrity and degeneration resulting in disease.

Consumption of any cooked or processed food, and exposure to pollution create toxicity, imbalances, and deficiencies. When enough toxicity accumulates, resulting in compound cellular damage and degeneration, disease develops. I present evidence on pages 153-158.

Chapter 3
How Much Toxicity Does It Take To Develop Disease And How Do We Reverse It?

We experience degenerative conditions and symptoms from accumulated toxins. For some people, a little toxicity is enough to create disease. In weaker individuals, often the mothers had not eaten a healthy diet and/or had been exposed to toxins, including medication and cleaning compounds. The toxins flowed from mothers' blood and accumulated in the fetuses.

Toxins must be dissolved and discarded. Tests have proved that the accumulations of the byproducts formed and released from dissolving or discarding toxins also must be isolated and removed. That isolation, dissolution, neutralization, secretion and excretion of toxins is called detoxification.

Symptoms, such as nausea, vomit, diarrhea, edema (swelling), failed appetite, insomnia, aches and pains, lethargy, impotence, weight-loss, colds, flu, fever, and even immobility are indications of detoxification. Detoxification is necessary to reverse disease. It is our bodies' way of cleansing themselves of toxins. Swelling occurs during periods when massive toxins inundate the blood and/or tissues, such as after injury including poison. Swelling is a sign of increased circulation required to dilute and remove toxins and to increase nutrients to toxic areas.

Healing follows detoxification. Proper healing is when the body reproduces cells to repopulate areas where toxins destroyed cells. Improper healing occurs when our bodies cannot reproduce cells because of deficiencies. Our bodies must relocate live or mummified cells (scar tissue) from other areas of our bodies when our cells cannot reproduce. That process weakens the entire body.

What are the nutrients for proper
detoxification and healing?

Chapter 4
Journey To Optimal Health

I tried many alternatives to medical therapies. The only alternative that was effective and long-lasting was a particular raw-food diet. Over many years, it completely reversed my cancers as well as my juvenile diabetes, psoriasis, angina, bursitis and developmental autism. I discovered that particular raw foods and particular raw-food combinations gradually reversed almost every disease 90% of the time as long as I did not accept medical therapies. Although sometimes I experienced reduction in symptoms, I observed less overall recovery when I used medication, medical therapies or dietary supplements. Medication, medical therapies and supplements often stop symptoms while they further compromise and/or destroy health. I will discuss this more on pages 159-161.

Empirical evidence proved to me that the health of an individual depends greatly on what she or he eats and how food is prepared and combined. The foods to eat depend on an individual's health-needs. Generally, each food affects the body differently because each food offers a different formula of nutrients. Because of our individual chemistry, some times the same food affects individuals differently.

Over a 33-year period, empirical and scientific evidence proved to me that raw, unheated, uncooked, non-irradiated, unprocessed food promotes and generates good health and well-being and reverses disease. Empirical and scientific evidence has proved that cooked and processed food promotes disease. I am one of thousands of people who can testify to those truths from experience. I realized that health-giving food is raw food that is suited for us anatomically and biochemically. I discuss which foods are suited for us on pages 151-153. To discover which foods reverse particular ailments and disease, read *The Primal Diet; We Want To Live, Volume 2.*

To see several hundred testimonials go to the website: www.PrimalDiet.com.

If you are interested in my journey and others' case histories of disease reversals with diet, and to discover specific foods that have proved to beneficially affect an individual's health, read *The Primal Diet; We Want To Live, Vol. 1.*

Chapter 5

Man's Dietary Origin;
Humans Lived Without Disease

All creatures in nature have thrived on the ability to grow, propagate, and live disease-free with the ingestion of raw food that is complete with particular combinations of enzymes, vitamins, minerals, proteins, fats, carbohydrates and many unidentified nutrients. Our bodies have evolved for millions of years digesting raw foods that are complete microcosms within themselves, resplendent in nutrients and bacteria.

The story that cavemen started a fire every time they ate is anthropological supposition. Anyone who has lived primitively, as I did for several years, knows that there are numerous conditions that prevent fire-making. Cavemen had to have eaten their meat diet mostly fireless. Prior to the importation of German cooking cauldrons, Eskimos ate their meat raw. Cavemen probably did, too. The Eskimo-diet was 99% animal products[2] (fish, Caribou, seal, moose, bear, whale, etc.). Eskimos lived free of degenerative diseases. Based on my experiences, eating <u>raw</u> food was the primary factor that enabled them to stay strong, energetic, and happy, and to live without disease under strenuous climatic conditions.

Why did we make the transition from eating raw animal foods to eating mainly grains and vegetables? The most plausible

---

[2] Throughout this book, when I state "animal products" or "animal food", I mean flesh food (meat and glands), eggs and dairy products. I do not mean food that is fed to animals.

explanation is that nomadic humans decided to settle in one place. They overpopulated and consumed most of the animal life around their dwellings. They had to eat something else. Rather than leave their homes, migrate to where more meat roamed and rebuild their villages, they found ways to utilize vegetation, legumes, nuts and grains. They learned that cooking allowed their digestive tracts to utilize more substances from grains, legumes and vegetables. Cooking, however, gradually caused health problems, including dehydration, constipation and severe sensitivity to hot and cold temperatures. Those problems gradually became innumerable ailments and diseases. I will discuss more about nutrients destroyed by cooking and processing on pages 153-157. More on disease and disease-free living is discussed on pages 164-186.

Chapter 6
Can We Digest Cooked And Processed Food?

Doctors and scientists have told people for a century that our bodies produce vitamins and enzymes to compensate for those destroyed by cooking and processing. They point to the fact that when people digest cooked food, pancreatic and stomach fluids show supplementation of nutrients destroyed by cooking. Because of that phenomenon, they conclude that it is healthy to eat cooked food. They have led us to believe that vitamins and enzymes spontaneously appear, as money grows on trees.

They have not told us that: 1) eating cooked food forces our pancreases to send hormonal and electromagnetic messages to every cell in our bodies, 2) those messages demand that nutrients be leeched from our cells to replace the nutrients lost during cooking and processing, 3) our cells sacrifice their innate high-quality supply of vitamins and enzymes to the functions of digestion, assimilation and utilization of cooked and processed food, 4) when our digestive systems are finished with those jobs, we suffer more leeching because our cells must send more nutrients to detoxify the poisons formed during cooking and processing, and 5) those leeching processes gradually and unnoticeably weaken every cell in our bodies. As a result, our entire bodies slowly deteriorate. Disease came quickly to those of us who were born weak and debilitated.

We must acknowledge that some people who eat cooked foods appear and feel healthy because they utilize cooked foods better than most people. Many people who eat cooked food, especially our youth, progressively deteriorate but do not realize it because they have great energy produced by hormones from overactive glands. That means they have an over-abundance of hormones. Much of the hormonal overproduction is from toxic junk food full of preservatives, pesticides, herbicides, fungicides, chemical fertilizers, hormones, antibiotics and other drugs fed to crops and animals we eat. Those hormones are often used by their bodies to replace the destroyed nutrients in cooked and processed food, to stimulate energy levels, and to mask illness-symptoms without eliminating disease. Many of those people's glands become too toxic, may harden later in life and/or become fatigued. Most often, those people do not realize they are diseased until it is too late to reverse their ill conditions easily. At that late stage, their glands do not produce enough hormones to carry on normal internal functions, much less utilize hormones as replacements for destroyed nutrients.

Can We Digest Raw Food?
In discussions over the years, approximately 30 doctors corroborated what Dr. Edinberg emphatically stated to me after he performed stomach surgery (vagotomy pyloroplasty): That I could not possibly digest properly because of that surgery. They all said that because I do not secrete hydrochloric acid for proper digestion, I must cook all food to get some value from it, even though cooking destroys much of the nutrient value that raw food supplies. Again, they terrorized me into believing them.

I followed their prescriptions and worsened to the extent that I was crippled. One cooked meat meal caused pustules to appear from my head to my waist, front and back. I noticed that if I did not eat cooked meat, I had fewer pimples. Every time I ate cooked or processed food, I felt side-effects; cooked meat affected me worst.

Using various diets, I experimented with myself first, then with animals and people. We found that raw food was, and is, the only food we digest thoroughly and properly with*out* carcinogenic toxins formed by cooking and side effects of those toxins.[3] How can doctors and scientists hold fast to their false beliefs and deny our testimony? How can they deny the quality of my health when their prognosis was that I would die horribly at least 34 years ago? How can they deny my healthy results from eating only raw food for the last 28 years? The answers to those questions are implied in the answers to these questions: Who funds research and who dictates the purpose of research? Could researchers be biased in favor of the economic gain from the pharmaceutical and food-processing industries? They use the example of a small portion of the population who live satisfactorily and even happily eating cooked food and taking their medications.

Researchers dictate what doctors believe. Most doctors, academia and the media, accept researchers' speculations as truth written in stone. People have been conditioned, in the name of "advanced" technological living, that anything "raw" or "primitive" is bad, and that technology at any price is good. The words "raw" and "primitive" have been propagandized to mean unclean, gross and disease-causing. The processed-food industry, with its well-paid scientists and marketers, and with government help from the USDA and FDA, blurred the meanings of the words "natural", "organic", "raw", and "uncooked". They have deliberately confused us about what truly gives to and takes away from our health. Empirical evidence proved erroneous the supposition that raw food is hard to digest and dangerous. Thousands of people and I are living examples that raw food digests and assimilates wonderfully.

It is true that most humans cannot properly digest the leaves, stalks and roots of whole raw vegetables, including seaweeds and dried algae. A human is not an herbivore. The key to digesting vegetation is to drink raw vegetable juices and eliminate the pulp. Raw vegetable juices are our best vitamin,

---

[3] Carcinogenic toxins discussed on pages 153-157.

enzyme and mineral supplements. More about our digestive abilities is on pages 151-153.

A diet of mainly raw meat, raw eggs and raw dairy proved to be safe, easily digested and the most nutritious.

Chapter 7
Should We Worry About Bacteria?

Bacterial concern is a phobia that has swept the "civilized" world. Our natural food-supply is being annihilated because of it. We must look rationally at the bacterial issue. Consider the fact that many tribes ate primarily unsalted raw meat, unsalted raw fats and/or unsalted raw dairy products from the beginning. They did not wash their hands or sterilize their food before eating. Every form of natural bacteria, including salmonella, E. coli and campylobacter[4] were eaten with their food, abundantly and constantly. Why were they vibrant, healthy and disease-free if microbes are the culprits?

From the time babies are born, they put everything in their mouths, dirt and microbes. It is believed that babies build immunity through small benign doses of bacteria, allergens, and pathogens. Some scientists call this "auto-immune inoculation". Rather than accept the inoculation-theory, I believe that for millions of years animals, including humans, formed working relationships with bacteria, including "pathogens". Those microbes have a janitorial role in nature and we benefit from them. When parents stop babies from putting stuff in their mouths, they hinder the relationship with microbes and the environment, unless of course the objects are poisonous, such as manmade chemicals and most toys.

---

[4] Three geneses of bacteria believed to cause food-poisoning. E.coli is found in bowels and feces and unscientifically presumed to cause death. More on pages 169-186.

Doctors told me that I was in danger of death from bacterial and parasitic food-poisoning. I was placed in the highest "at-risk" category. They terrorized me into believing that raw food with all of its bacteria would kill me. They were adamant about it. What they told me to eat did not work.

From desperation, I tried eating raw meats. Thousands of times, I ate raw meats and raw milk that were "microbe-infected" during my 32 years of experimentation and everyday-life. According to the assumptions of the medical and scientific communities, I should have suffered bacterial or parasitic food-poisoning thousands of times. I did not. Not once. Thousands of other "at-risk" individuals who switched to eating raw animal products to reverse their diseases and/or to improve their health also did not get sick.

I learned that the occurrence of diarrhea and vomit in people who ate raw food was less frequent than in people who ate cooked and processed food. I learned that in either case, bacteria were found. I discovered in studies of diarrhea and vomit that more often there were higher concentrations of bacteria in people who ate cooked food than in people who ate raw food. How, then, can the medical and scientific communities adhere to the belief that raw food causes bacterial food-poisoning? Their belief is based in fear, with no more rationale than the belief in evil spirits that motivated the witch hunts of medieval times.

Possible metabolic and environmental sources of vomit and diarrhea must be explored where "pathogens"[5] are found. These questions must be asked: Are pathogens the cause or the result of degenerative disease? Are they the cause or the cure? Is pointing the finger at microbes a distraction from the causes of disease? Is the pollution of our food, water and air predominantly the cause of diseases that include vomit and diarrhea? Are doctors and scientists using microbes as scapegoats for the causes of diseases that we create with our processing, medical therapies and pollution? All hypotheses

[5] Believed to be agents capable of producing disease. "Pathogen" is the medical term for "the bad guys". However, in reality, "pathogens" have a beneficial purpose.

must be explored by independent testing. Researchers must be held accountable to uphold the rules of evidence without the influence of special interests.

It is wise to know the myths as well as the truths regarding food in our time. Then we will be free to eat with peace of mind, joy and sensuality. Do not look to the medical or scientific communities for information on raw food. They have been prejudiced against it and know very little or nothing about raw food. They study and experiment with drugs, cooked and processed food. Although most make adamant claims against raw food, especially raw meats, they know little or nothing about the effects of raw food on health. I have met hundreds of doctors. Not one had any experience utilizing a raw-meat diet. I present more evidence on the myths and truths regarding bacteria on pages 169-186.

Chapter 8
What's Healthiest To Eat, And What's Not?

In an ideal world, a recipe for health satisfies a person's well-being and desire for good taste. In the natural world without pollution, animals are guided by instinct to eat raw food rich in nutrients and bacteria. They are guided by their senses. If we were healthy animals that allowed pure natural instinct to direct our sense of hunger, we would eat what is best for our bodily functions. Unfortunately, in our industrial-food, carbohydrate-addicted, bacterial-phobic society, we eat from the muddled combination of instinct, habituation and addiction.

I have observed and counseled many people who ate a raw instinctive diet. I tried and enjoyed a raw instinctive diet for six years. We ate only foods that appealed to our senses of smell, taste and fullness. We ate a lot of fruit because sweetness appealed to all of us. Even though we felt better in general, too often we suffered severe symptoms, over-emotionality, hyperactivity and irritability. Those experiences were no different than our experiences on the standard-American diet

(SAD). We assumed that instinctive-eating was a better diet because it was natural. When my teeth began to rapidly decay, I began to doubt the power of food. Someone suggested that I eat a modified raw diet that restricted high-carbohydrate food, including carrot and sweet-fruit juices, and sweet fruit. I was appalled at the suggestion because I loved sweet fruit.

Since I wanted to stop my tooth-decay, I tried eating a raw diet of meat, dairy, eggs, green vegetable juices and only ½ cup of fruit daily. The diet was not as enjoyable and I was often nauseated for the first 3 weeks but my life gradually improved. My tremendous anxiety over the polluted, greed-driven and fearful structure of society and government settled. I spent more time finding or creating solutions and less time brooding and being ineffective. I became less sensitive to cold temperatures and less hyperactive. My over-enthusiasm and zealousness mellowed. I became better able to communicate, write and read. When I ate too much fruit, I relapsed into heightened anxiety.

After a year of eating that way, I advised changes to my clients' diets. Some clients gradually experienced the same improvements that I had. Most of them experienced immediate improvements. It was a wonderful leap of progress toward a healthier, happier, disease-free life. I experimented with fine-tuning the diet. I continually found that raw fats, especially unsalted raw butter, are the primary substances that dissolve and bind with toxicity, protect our cells, reverse the greatest number and most severe cases of diseases, and deliver the greatest strength and energy. In an ideal healthy world, we would not need such an abundance of fat. In our civilized, polluted, disease-ridden world, we need an abundance of fat.

Before my move away from high-carbohydrate food, I discovered that most people do not regenerate cells to reverse or prevent the aging process of deterioration and disease without eating plenty of raw meat in combination with raw fats. My experience contradicted the conditioned-thinking that meats and fats are bad and cause obesity and a myriad of other diseases. After my shift away from eating high-carbohydrate food, I discovered that I healed more quickly. My clients who implemented the changes of diet also healed more quickly.

It was not long after my introduction to raw food that I became aware that our bodies have innumerable chores to complete every minute. They eat, digest, transport, utilize and assimilate food to energize, lubricate membranes, regenerate and reproduce to replace dead cells. Dead cells must be collected, transported, dissolved or disassembled, sorted through for usable substances, and the byproducts discarded. The innumerable enzymes and vitamins found in raw food are the helpers necessary to accomplish those tasks. When we eat raw food, we have trillions of helpers to accomplish all of those tasks with little waste.

When we cook and/or process our food, we massacre our helpers, causing our bodies to have to do all of the chores on their own. Cooking and processing exhaust our bodies' natural resources. We further exhaust our natural resources trying to clean up the toxicity after the massacre. The pancreas must produce and discharge extra hormones and electromagnetic signals that leech quality vitamins, enzymes, minerals, fats, proteins, and carbohydrates from every cell to clean up the massacre, as well as continue to perform all of its ordinary, innumerable bodily tasks. In most people, many years of leeching causes gradual but marked decrease in strength and agility. That is common in our society. Leeching reduces the ability of each and every cell to withstand the increased toxicity that accompanies this process and produces diseases of all kinds.

A simple analogy is this: We are the mayors of a city (the body) in which we live. We must renovate, maintain and keep the city efficient and clean. Our enzymes are the maids, gardeners, food-preparers, handy and craft persons, helpers and managers that accomplish all of the chores necessary every second. If we massacre the workers (cook and/or process our food, destroying enzymes and vitamins), not only do we have to clean the massacre, we must seize workers from other tasks to do all of the chores of the city. That depletes our resources and depresses the population (our cells). That entire process is impossible to maintain. We cannot properly accomplish the chores. Pollution collects and creates a toxic environment within the city and the city deteriorates.

Taking the analogy another step, let's say we built New York City (our body) from poor and poisonous materials (cooked and processed foods). The city-dwellers, animals and plants (our cells and microbes) are variously affected. They overproduce waste because they are weak and lack the resources necessary to maintain a self-sustainable environment. Grime accumulates in the homes, buildings, streets, fields, parks and skies, deteriorating structures and life. Now let's say we become aware that we built a polluted and rapidly deteriorating, diseased city. How much time will it take to reorganize, demolish faulty structures, load, transport and bury waste, neutralize poisonous matter, search for and gather nutrients, negotiate, redesign, renovate and restructure? How long will roads be blocked and over-congested? What degree of inconvenience, pollution and pain will residents and workers suffer? If people had to completely rebuild New York City, how long would it take? Two hundred years? Five hundred?

Our bodies do not normally sustain a complete, instant cataclysmic breakdown of organs, glands or systems as New York City did when the Twin Towers collapsed. The body has to take itself apart bit by bit. Bacteria, molds and parasites help speed the process by consuming the weak or dead cells and degenerative tissue, reducing them to lesser wastes. Viruses are not alive. They are solvents (soaps that dissolve) produced within cells to dissolve toxicity, including degenerative cells. It is cellular self-surgery. The detoxification process is slow, accompanied by many uncomfortable symptoms.

The work of doctors Pottenger and Howell corroborates the results of my observations of more than 5,000 people who eat a mainly raw diet. Our conclusion is that animals require 5 generations to reach optimal health. Since bones in humans take approximately 7½ years to be completely replaced one time, our bodies require approximately 40 years to rebuild themselves to reach optimal health. Fortunately, we do not have to wait for a pot of gold at the end of the rainbow to feel better. We improve every year on a health-giving diet. (I outline more on health-giving foods, food-combining and daily dietary plans on pages 26-43.)

Sleep And Healing

Ninety-percent of healing that is regeneration and cellular reproduction occurs during sleep and very restful states. Naps are health-giving, especially when feeling sleepy or tired. A 10- to 60-minute nap often does wonders for the body, mind and spirit.

People who are sleepy, need sleep. Getting well and strong depends on lots of sleep. As we get healthier and stronger, we need less sleep. When I was recovering from cancer, especially cancer treatments, I slept 12-20 hours each day. Now, on the average, I sleep 4½ -5 hours each day. I enjoy excellent clarity and stamina in my wakeful hours. Two to six days each month, I may sleep 6-8 hours. I usually take a 10-60 minute nap everyday.

Bowel Movements

The number and volume of bowel movements depends on the food, health of intestinal bacteria and amount of toxins that enter the bowels. One movement every 1 to 3 days may be appropriate for one individual while 5 movements in a single day may be appropriate for another individual. Frequency, volume and consistency naturally vary and should not be a concern unless there is considerable discomfort. If constipation is a problem, I suggest that you eat more unsalted raw butter. Also, see pages 148-150.

Volume Two

**The Recipe For Healthy Living
& Optimal Recipes!**

Chapter 9
Delicious Is In The Palate Of The Masticator

You may have noticed that the same products of processed and cooked foods taste exactly the same, package after package and bottle after bottle. Processing and cooking destroy the naturally occurring flavor-nutrients in food. Food often becomes bitter and unappealing. Food-manufacturers must season the food to make it appealing and habit-forming. Often, a bite of cooked and processed food loses flavor and palatability within five or six chews, unless it has been heavily salted, chemically flavored or seasoned. Because processed and cooked foods do not satisfy our nutritive needs and cause extreme toxicity, our bodies are always unsatisfied and starving, regardless of how full we feel. One of two extreme symptoms is often the result: 1) over-eating or 2) lack of appetite.

Most processed foods are made from spoiled, rancid, and repulsive-tasting fruit, vegetable, grain, or animal products. For example, most commercial tomato sauces and tomato soups are made with spoiled tomatoes. They are full of fermentation and molds. The tomatoes sit in open trucks in the hot sun for days, spoiling. After the spoiled tomatoes are sterilized, they are seasoned with chemical and/or processed flavorings to hide the rotten taste. If we eat those sauces and soups, we eat rotten food and chemicals.

A little spoiled raw food has been shown to be beneficial to health, but not when processed, sterilized and eaten repeatedly. Diets of spoiled, cooked and processed foods have proved repeatedly to coincide with disease. We may pay twice more for them, through loss of health and work.

Fresh raw foods usually have delightful tastes. Some of us have retained a degree of our natural taste instincts and easily appreciate meaty raw foods. However, most of us live in palatal conflict. We crave foods that are not good for us. I vowed to resolve that conflict. I offer health-giving raw recipes that have assisted many people with varied food preferences toward achieving optimal health and reversing disease.

Each raw food tastes uniquely different, especially if it comes from heirloom seed, rather than hybrid. One tomato may taste slightly different from another tomato from the same vine. Therefore, each time a raw-food recipe is prepared, it will have a somewhat different flavor. This is the ultimate dietary variety, the spice of life.

For some people, eating raw meat is nearly impossible unless it has a familiar flavor. Therefore, most of the recipes I present in this book are to increase peoples' appetite for raw meat. When I refer to raw meat, I mean flesh food, whether it is seafood, fish, fowl, beef, sheep, venison, buffalo, pork or wild meat. Other recipes, such as raw cheesecakes, are wonderfully delicious, raw, health-giving sweet meals.

All recipes in this book promote better health when included in a balanced diet. To discover what a balanced diet is for each individual, read *The Primal Diet; We Want To Live, Vols. 1 & 2*. I suggested two general dietary plans in this book, pages 40-41.

Chapter 10
The Best Health-Giving Raw Food

- **Honey, bee pollen and royal jelly should not be artificially heated above 93° F (33° C), nor stored below 45° F (7° C).**
- **Fats should not be artificially heated above 96° F (35° C) nor stored below 38° F (2° C), except olive oil, which should not be stored below 50° F (10° C).**

- Milk and milk products should not be artificially heated above 98° F nor stored below 45° F (7° C).
- Meats should not be artificially heated above 98° F (37° C) nor stored below 38° F (2° C).
- Eggs should not be artificially heated above 98° F (37° C) nor stored below 68° F (20° C). Eggs lose many nutrients when refrigerated. Eggs should not be refrigerated except when a recipe calls for it. Recipes that contain egg should not be refrigerated after being prepared. Most recipes will last for 24 hours outside of refrigeration.
- Other foods should not be artificially heated above 104° F (39° C) nor stored below 45° F (7° C).

Following are the foods that have been proved to assimilate well in human digestion and are able to be properly utilized for balance, growth, regeneration, cellular reproduction and lubrication, soothing, calming, cleansing and fueling.

RAW EGGS, Free-Range, are one of the best compact foods in nature. Eggs are the ultimate complete fast-food. However, the protein in eggs is not utilized for cellular reproduction. They are utilized for regeneration and maintenance and cannot be substituted for meat except occasionally. The relationship between raw eggs and salmonella-poisoning is a myth.[6]

Eggs are remarkable for everyone, especially those who are infirm. Three years ago, a medical doctor called me on a Thursday evening about her 70-year-old female patient with emphysema. She explained that her patient had been mainly bedridden for 2 years, was on 100% oxygen and respiratory machines. She prognosed that her patient would die that weekend unless I could help. I told her that the only thing that I thought might help at that late stage was eggs. I recommended that she get her patient 10 dozen raw eggs and put them on her bed-table. I suggested that she ask her patient to eat one as often as she could and that there was no limit. Very early Monday morning, I received a call from the patient. She told me that she

---

[6] *The Great Egg Panic* by Emily Green, LA Times, Jan. 4, 2000.

was off the machines, out of bed and feeling stronger than she had in years. She had eaten 66 eggs over the weekend.

If eggs are whipped, beaten or blenderized without milk, cream or coconut cream, many of the enzymes are oxidized and lost. Therefore, if we eat eggs alone, do not mix, beat, whip or blenderize them. Many clients enjoy sucking them from the shell, as I do, by poking a whole at each end. Hold the head back and suck. Be certain to put a finger over the bottom hole when your head returns to normal position or egg will drain. Others enjoy eating eggs Rocky-style, that is, broken into a glass and consumed without any other food, not whipped, beaten or mixed. For those who are squeamish about the texture, sipping and swallowing the egg white makes eating eggs Rocky-style very easy and non-repulsive.

RAW FAT is the most utilized nutrient in our bodies, especially in our toxic industrial world. It helps stabilize and relax the body markedly when in combination with raw meat. Fats help white blood-cell production, assist microbial activity and provide for lubricants to accomplish a variety of functions. Lubricants facilitate movement without frictional deterioration, protect cells from heat, cold and caustic substances, provide hormones to regulate activity, and, when acting in conjunction with 15% protein and 5% alcohol formed internally from carbohydrate, fats dissolve all sorts of toxic substances. Fats provide the greatest, strongest and most efficient energy possible.

Before modern man encroached upon native populations, such as the Eskimo, Masai, Fulani and Samburu, natives consumed fat as 40-60% of their caloric intake. The Eskimo endured the coldest temperatures. The Masai, Fulani and Samburu tribes in Africa endured very hot temperatures. The Eskimo, Masai, Fulani and Samburu did not suffer any heart maladies as long as they ate their natural diet of raw meat and raw fat, absent of sugar and cooked starches.

RAW MEAT provides easily used proteins to build, rebuild, regenerate, and reproduce cells throughout the body. I have observed that raw meat is the only protein that facilitates nerve-tissue regeneration and cellular reproduction. Although all meats help regenerate every type of cell, particular raw meats more readily help the regeneration of certain types of cells. Red meat, such as beef, buffalo, venison, lamb, etc., helps regenerate and develop most glandular tissue, blood and muscle. White meat such as chicken, turkey and other fowl, helps build and regenerate connective tissue, nerves, lymph, skin, and tissue in general. White meat such as nonfarmed, ocean wild-caught fish and seafood, helps reconstitute nerves, including the brain. I have seen that eating 1-3 pounds of raw meat daily helps regenerate, heal the body, and reverse the common toxic deterioration associated with aging and disease. Regarding the ratio of red and white meat to eat for each individual, see *The Primal Diet; We Want To Live*, Appendix P.

I recommend only ocean wild-caught raw fish, not farmed, except oysters, clams and scallops. I suggest all varieties including Swordfish, which has the highest mercury content. When digested and made bioactive by plankton and eaten by fish, traces of mercury are great detoxifiers of toxic mercury in the body. Bioactive and non-cauterized mercury in raw fish helps buoyancy of fish. When fish are cooked, mercury and other metallic minerals become free-radicals and toxic.

I have noted in my clients, a continual rise in nausea and vomit from eating freshwater fish, especially freshwater-caught salmon, catfish and sturgeon. Freshwater fish have a greater number of toxins because our fresh waters are approximately 30% polluted. Our oceans are approximately 4% polluted. I do not eat freshwater fish unless I catch it in a non-polluted lake. There are very few non-polluted lakes left in the USA because of the pollution created by water-sport vehicles, agricultural chemicals, and agricultural and mining waste.

Eating organic glands is recommended in all cases, especially Chronic Fatigue Syndrome, Fibromyalgia and Lupus. To make glands palatable, I created POWER DRINKS; pages 103-104.

When deciding on cuts of meat to eat, consider that all hunter tribes discard the tender meats, or feed them to the elderly. They have experienced that eating tender meat causes weakened cells. The-tougher-the-meat-the-better is their motto.

FRESH, RAW, NON-PASTEURIZED, NON-IRRADIATED GREEN VEGETABLE JUICES are important for optimal health because they are the only nontoxic vitamin, enzyme and mineral supplements. Vegetable juices replace the vitamins, enzymes and minerals that are lost in daily activity. They provide for the management of toxicity from years of eating cooked food. They provide for proper blood alkalinity without alkalinizing the acidic parts of our digestive tract.

Because we are constantly in accelerated detoxification due to our toxic conditions, our blood tends to be too acidic with waste compounds. That acidic blood-condition often causes cravings for too much fruit and cooked starches, lethargy, irritability, repulsion toward meats, and anorexia. Drinking green vegetable juices 2-4 times a day, but not in combination with other foods, helps to neutralize the acidic compounds in the blood. They do not over-alkalinize the intestines. Most often, they eliminate the symptoms listed above. Drinking green vegetable juices daily ensures the replacement of the enzymes, vitamins and minerals that are lost because of deficient soils, reduced through the stress of food transport from the field to our dinner plates, and that have been leeched from our bodies from years of eating cooked foods. Several juice recipes appear on pages 54-56.

High-carbohydrate vegetable juices, such as root vegetables (carrot, beet, potato and yam) raise the blood-sugar level too high, making us overly emotional. Often the blood-sugar level soars and then drops, leaving us mentally and emotionally fatigued, sleepy, irritable and/or depressed. Therefore, it is important to restrict the quantity of high-carbohydrate vegetable juices. Most often, I suggest that a vegetable drink contain no more than 10% carrot juice.

Since the USDA and FDA have worked against our health and acted in favor of agribusinesses, they have ruined the true meaning of organic. Now, even organic produce may contain agricultural chemicals. To help prevent agricultural chemicals from damaging our health, it would be best to put ½ teaspoon of sun-dried clay into each quart of vegetable juices. The clay will absorb most, if not all, of the toxins that may be found in the juices. Prior to use, mix clay with water and let stand for 5 days.

UNHEATED HONEY contains an insulin-like substance that is produced by bees when collecting nectar. That insulin-like substance converts 90% of the carbohydrate in nectar into enzymes that help digest, assimilate and utilize protein. Unheated honey is a wonderful sweet food that helps digest all types of meat. That honey is wonderful for infants, fed in small amounts at a time.

The insulin-like substance begins detrimental alteration at 93° F (33° C) and is destroyed at 100° F (37° C). Diabetics, hypoglycemics and some infants cannot utilize honey if the insulin-like substance is destroyed. Honey that is heated above 104° F (39° C) is radical sugar that often causes slow deterioration of membranes in the body. Honey heated above 104° F (39° C) may cause toxicity in some infants.

CARBOHYDRATES are required for only 5% of the optimal diet for humans. They are needed to properly utilize fat for energy and make solvents for cleansing. The best sources for carbohydrates are green vegetable juices and a small amount of fruit. When we eat too much carbohydrate, we create many conditions that diminish health. Carbohydrates such as root vegetables, grains, nuts and seeds, and products made from them, such as pasta, cereals, cakes, donuts, pancakes, breads and cookies create health problems.

For example, after white man brought native people processed and cooked breads, sugar and alcohol, natives developed all of the diseases that "civilized" mankind suffers, including cavities, diabetes, osteoporosis, and cancer. Archeologists have concluded that as Native Americans hunted less, while gathering and cultivating more nuts, grains and fruit, they developed osteoporosis and dental decay. It seems that all races are unable to properly eliminate carbohydrate wastes.

Some carbohydrate wastes are called glycotoxins. One glycotoxin, termed Advanced Glycation End-products (AGEs), was studied at Columbia University's Department of Medicine. Researchers found that AGEs store in a healthy body at a rate of 70%, and in an unhealthy body at a rate of 90%.[7] AGEs contaminate the body and predispose it to cancer and molds such as candida and other yeast infections.

If most people eat too much carbohydrate, the blood-fat level drops, the blood-sugar level soars, and the pancreas overworks to regulate the sugar level. That often results in manic behavior and hyperactivity. Then that energy drops quickly and leaves us mentally and emotionally fatigued, irritable, sleepy and/or depressed. As happens with processed sweets, I have seen that eating too much fruit or carrot juice causes many people to become overly emotional. That is similar to monkeys who live on fruit.

In this modern age, several factors are responsible for people eating mainly grain products (bread, pasta, cereal, etc.) and vegetables. Grain products are less expensive than meat, eggs and dairy, and we are told that red meat, eggs and dairy cause disease. Advertising campaigns from the processed-food industry have contributed to the propaganda that blames fats and meats in general for many diseases.

Contrarily, fat-free diets have caused a startling increase in degenerative diseases in the past two decades, according to Harvard University. Non-meat diets slow healing and regeneration. For humans, a raw diet that is very low in carbohydrate has proved to produce a disease-free, happy life.

A LITTLE FRUIT eaten with raw fat slows fruit-sugar digestion and helps to prevent manic, hyperactive, irritable and/or depressive reactions. To avoid those reactions, I suggest

---

[7] *Cellular Receptors for Advanced Glycation End Products; Implications for Induction of Oxidant Stress and Cellular Dysfunction in the Pathogenesis of Vascular Lesions*, Schmidt, Hori, Brett, Du Yan, Wautier, Stern; Review, Arteriosclerosis and Thrombosis, 1994, Vol. 14, (10):1521-8.

eating the whole fruit (except citrus rind) and rarely, or never, consume fruit juices. For people with diabetes and glycemic conditions, I recommend no more than 4-7 ounces of fruit, depending on a person's size, once every 2-3 days. As I stated, high-carbohydrate fruit should always be eaten with a raw fat, such as raw cream, raw coconut cream, unsalted raw butter, avocado, or a combination of unsalted raw butter and no-salt-added raw cheese.

Too much fruit causes over emotionality because it causes low blood-protein and blood-fat levels, disrupts the sugar levels, irritates tissue, and leeches fats from the nervous system, causing lesions in the myelin. Some people should not eat fruit except on rare occasions, such as bulimics and diabetics, and when they do, they should always eat high-carbohydrate fruit with an equal amount of fat. Fruit also causes edema (water retention). I have met 8 people of 2,300 who were able to maintain health and eat a high-carbohydrate fruit diet without ill symptoms. If you do not get overly emotional or manic within 24 hours after eating fruit, more fruit might be fine for you.

NUTS, when eaten plain and/or in quantity and/or too often, cause carbohydrate toxicity. Raw nuts contain enzyme inhibitors that prevent proper protein digestion and cause mineral loss. I created the NUT FORMULA that neutralizes the enzyme inhibitors in nuts. The Nut Formula should be eaten only once or twice a week to satisfy needs and eliminate cravings for breads, pastas, cakes, donuts, rice, etc. It helps harness and detoxify neurological toxins. If consumed more often, especially two days in a row, it can cause neurological detoxification that will interfere with sleep between 12:30 and 5:30 A.M. Eating nuts that are not in combination with all of the foods in the Nut Formula, often interferes with protein-digestion of any food consumed within 48 hours after eating nuts. That can make sleep at certain hours difficult.

See Nut Formula, page 117, to learn the foods to combine with raw nuts so that they help create health rather than interfere with health.

OILS, such as olive and flax are 90% solvent-reactive. That is, they are mainly used as cleansers to dissolve toxins. Our bodies cannot easily utilize pressed oils for lubrication, relaxation and stabilization. Pressed oils are beneficial in dissolving internal adhesions (scars) and dead cells, including benign or malignant tumors, and arterial and lymphatic congestion and plaque. Pressed oils often cause dry and acrid conditions in the body. I recommend the moderate eating of oils, no more than once a day or every other day, and that oils be consumed mainly with one meat meal. The body uses coconut cream the same as it does olive and flax oils but without drying the body because coconut cream can lubricate and soothe. Coconut cream is better.

In WW I, a Russian general recorded in his log that 3 months after his troops exhausted the raw butter supply and resorted to consuming olive oil, the men's hair, nails and skin dried. The log stated that several weeks after they were able to obtain raw dairy again, the men's hair, nails and skin became supple and moist.

Olive oil should never be refrigerated. Flax oil and coconut cream should always be refrigerated. As of this publication, only olive and flax oils are pressed below 96° F (36° C) and have not been solvent extracted. Absolutely no coconut oil or butter is produced under 118° F (46° C), no matter what the labels claim.

WATER that is not in raw food has no active ions, electrolytes nor minerals bound with nutrients. It must have all 3 properties or it is only 10% cellularly utilizable. Water leeches nutrients from our blood and intestines, and dilutes digestive juices so that when we eat, we do not digest or assimilate our food properly or efficiently. That leeching often causes wastes to embed in body-tissue rather than being discarded from the body.

It is a false notion that water nurtures and hydrates tissue. In fact, water dries the cells while it bloats the body because 90% of it circulates in the blood serum without cellular absorption. That also applies to the H_2O in cooked food. People who eat cooked food cannot absorb much of the H_2O into their cells. Their cells become dehydrated.

Most people who consume cooked and processed food, processed drinks and water, evaporate 2 quarts of water during the night. Most people who consume live raw food including meat, milk and vegetable juices may evaporate only 2 pints throughout the night after they have been on this Primal Diet for several years. Water is never a good replacement for body fluids spent during evaporation/perspiration because cells cannot absorb it. Only H_2O that is nutrient bound in food properly replaces fluids.

People believe that water lubricates the body. How can water lubricate anything? Fats lubricate. Try lubricating devices with water and they will disintegrate. Water disintegrates soil and rock so that plants can eat those particles. Drinking vast quantities of water also disintegrates the human body, causing frequent urination, a sense of being too cold in temperatures as high as 70° F (21° C), weight-loss in many people and bloating in many others.

Raw food contains from 55% to 92% H_2O that is 92-100% cellularly utilizable. Dehydration is impossible on the Primal Diet when water is not consumed. I drink about 1 cup of water per week without exercise. I may drink a little more if involved in physical activity. I recommend that people drink raw milk and green vegetable juices and eat tomatoes to fill their H_2O requirements. Most often, eating raw tomatoes and raw fat satisfies thirst and dryness, including dry mouth, better than other foods. When physically active, I drink 2 quarts of raw milk, 1-2 tomatoes and up to 1 1/2 quarts of green vegetable juices per day that are all rich with nutrients to completely satisfy my H_2O needs. To satisfy dry mouth and severe thirst, I consume butter and/or cream. Rather than dehydrated, we are delipidated. That means we are deficient in the raw fats that can properly lubricate us. Our thirst is more for raw fat than for H_2O.

Chapter 11
FOOD-COMBINING
For Proper Digestion And Assimilation

Combining acidic and alkaline foods often neutralizes digestibility, resulting in toxins that deprive us of nutrients.

VEGETABLES and vegetable juices are alkalinizing and require an alkaline digestive environment for proper digestion. Except in small amounts as flavoring, vegetables and vegetable juices should not be eaten or drunk with acidic foods. Bland fruits, such as tomato and avocado are not vegetables and may be eaten with acidic or alkaline foods.

MEAT, EGGS, MILK, CHEESE, NUTS and SEEDS require an acidic digestive environment for proper digestion.

UNSALTED RAW BUTTER, RAW CREAM, AND UNHEATED COCONUT CREAM are neutral and may be consumed with either acidic or alkaline foods.

RAW MILK requires an acidic digestive environment for proper digestion. It may be consumed at any time except within an hour before or an hour after vegetable juices. For speedier healing, I suggest that we do not drink so much milk that we cancel our appetite for meat and other foods. If we experience discomfort after drinking raw milk with other foods, it would be better to drink raw milk alone. Drinking raw milk that has warmed to room temperature for at least 5 hours aids digestion. When milk is drunk cold from refrigeration, milk proteins and sugars may pass into the blood undigested and cause allergic reactions. If I drink cold milk from the refrigerator, I experience stomach cramps and sometimes cramps in my hands and feet.

Concerning Vegetable Juices
- Wait at least one hour after drinking vegetable juices before eating or drinking any other food, except unsalted raw butter, raw cream, unheated coconut cream, and unheated honey.

- Wait at least one hour after eating or drinking any other food before drinking vegetable juices, except unsalted raw butter, raw cream, and unheated coconut cream, and unheated honey.

Concerning Whole Vegetables (Salads)
- Rarely should we eat whole vegetables but when we do, vegetables should not be eaten sooner than 1 hour after any other food.
- Vegetables move through the intestines slowly. Acidic foods will catch up with them and interfere with digestion. Therefore, no other food should be eaten within 5 hours after eating a vegetable salad.

Concerning Fruits
- If experiencing tooth or gum sensitivity or pain in a particular area, do not eat high-carbohydrate fruits, especially apples and citrus.
- Alkaline fruits, such as bananas, peaches and figs, should not be consumed more than once a day, and should not be consumed with meat. They should be eaten with coconut cream, coconut, avocado, unsalted raw butter, raw cream, no-salt-added raw cheese or occasionally raw eggs.
- Acidic fruits, such as lemon, lime, pineapple and tangerine, may be consumed with fowl or fish when in combination with an added fat, such as raw cream, unsalted raw butter, no-salt-added raw cheese, coconut cream, coconut or avocado.

Concerning Meats
- Combining alkaline or acidic fruits with red meats usually turns too much of the protein into fuel or solvents. That reduces healing and obstructs the reversal of the aging process. The combination is not harmful but can hinder the healing processes and instigate too much detoxification. There is an exception: A little acidic fruit, such as lemon, lime, pineapple and apple cider vinegar, may be mixed or blended with fat 10 minutes prior to combining with red meat. Example: Tartar sauce eaten with red meat.

Concerning Cheese
- Combine cheese with at least an equal amount of fat, especially butter, to prevent constipation.

Chapter 12
An Optimal Diet

The Recipe For Removing Deep-Tissue Toxicity

On the Primal Diet, it is very important to gain and lose weight to remove imbedded toxicity. Without excess fat, the body cannot afford to make solvents, dissolve toxicity, neutralize, harness and contain it. Low body-fat levels only allow for basal metabolism and no deep cleansing. Most diseases are caused by concentrations of embedded toxicity. When a person lacks fat reserve, any toxin that enters the body or is loosed will cause cellular damage. They will be absorbed into cells. When a body has fat-reserves, toxins are collected and absorbed into fat, where they do little harm.

How many thin people do we know who are calm? How many thin people do we know who are hyperactive, physically and/or emotionally intense, easily irritated, manic, short-fused, and never satisfied? How many who are overweight? Physically, raw fat and happy is more often true. Our idea about thin should be refashioned until we become healthy. Now, fat is beautiful.

I recommend that men gain 15-30 pounds and women 12-15 pounds above what should be their normal weight (not according to thin-fashion). The excess weight should be achieved within two months. It should be maintained for another 2 months. That allows the body to utilize the stored fats as solvents to withdraw toxins from deep tissue and dissolve them. Then, it is time to eat the weight-loss diet to remove the toxin-filled excess fats. The process is similar to an oil-change in machinery. When the oil becomes black and thick with waste, it is time to change it. For the human body, I found that the cycle is best employed twice yearly. That vastly reduced symptoms of detoxification when detoxification occurred.

Some people have been able to gain the excess weight in as little as 10 days but it is important to hold it for at least 8 weeks. Some people require 2 weeks and some 3 months to lose the excess weight on the suggested weight-loss program on page 42.

The time required for weight-gain and weight-loss is individual. Two wardrobes are needed: 1) trim, not thin, and 2) oversized. Women should gain at least two sizes larger than their trim size. Men and women, get a temporary belly; it is healthier on and off!

I created the following paradigm from 35 years of experience, experimentation and research. An optimal diet consists of all organically grown food and generally contains:

Daily Intake:*

* 4-6 ounces only of raw fruit with equal amounts of raw fat consumed midday. Raw fruit should not be more than 5% of our total food consumption.
* 1-3 pounds (3-9 cups) of raw meat (red meat, and/or seafood, and/or fowl). Raw meat should be 25 to 30% of our diet.
* 8-24 ounces of raw fat (unsalted butter, cream, coconut cream juiced from coconut, meat, eggs, unsalted cheese, coconut, avocado, oils cold-pressed below 96° F (35° C)). Raw fat should be 25% of our diet.
* 2-6 cups of raw green vegetable juices. Green vegetable juices should be 25 to 30% of our diet.
* 8-12 ounces raw milk. Raw milk should be 10 to 20% of our diet. If we are active or athletic, 1-2 quarts raw milk may be consumed and plenty of butter to satisfy our sense of thirst. If milk is not available, the proportion of other foods increases, especially vegetable juices and butter.
* Salad may be eaten once every 2 to 4 weeks, or not at all. It would be better for digestion if that salad, if eaten, were eaten as the last food of that day. Whole vegetable salads often cause constipation on a raw diet by neutralizing acidic bacteria responsible for forming stools in the bowels and by interfering with digestion of other food. Usually, vegetable juices provide every thing we need from vegetables.

---

* Measurements: Meats are by weight in ounces and pounds; all other foods are by volume in teaspoons, tablespoons, ounces, cups, pints, etc. Percentages are by volume of food, not by weight.

General Daily Eating Schedule Recommendations #1
(This plan consists of three meat meals daily and is better for people with slower metabolism, lethargy and glycemic problems, including diabetes.)

- After waking, drink 4-12 ounces green vegetable juices.
- 45-60 minutes later, eat 6-10 ounces (1-2 cups) raw meat with raw egg(s) and/or 2-5 tablespoons raw butter, raw cream, raw coconut cream, no-salt-added raw cheese with equal amount of butter or avocado. One or a combination of several raw fats may be eaten at a meal, such as in a sauce.
- Next, 45-90 minutes later, drink a blended milkshake consisting of 1-4 raw eggs, 3-6 ounces raw milk, 1-4 ounces raw cream and 1-2 tablespoons unheated honey.
- At least 1 hour later, drink another 4-12 ounces green vegetable juices.
- At least 1 hour later, eat 6-10 ounces (1-2 cups) raw meat with raw egg(s) and/or 2-5 tablespoons raw butter, raw cream, raw coconut cream, no-salt-added raw cheese with an equal amount of butter or avocado. One or a combination of several raw fats may be eaten at a meal, such as in a sauce.
- 60-90 minutes later, eat 4-6 ounces fruit with 3-6 ounces of either raw cream, raw coconut cream, raw butter or avocado. You may combine any or all of the above, or you may drink another milkshake without fruit.
- At least 1 hour later, drink another 4-12 ounces green vegetable juices.
- At least 1 hour later, eat 6-10 ounces (1-2 cups) raw meat with raw egg(s) and/or 2-5 tablespoons raw butter, raw cream, raw coconut cream, no-salt-added raw cheese with an equal amount of butter or avocado. One or a combination of several raw fats may be eaten at a meal, such as in a sauce.
- 45-90 minutes later, drink a blended Moisturizing/ Lubrication Formula; page 146.
- At least 1 hour later, drink another 4-12 ounces green vegetable juices.

General Daily Eating Schedule Recommendations #2
(This plan consists of two meat meals daily and is better for people with high metabolism and hyperactivity.):

- **After waking, drink 4-12 ounces green vegetable juices.**
- **45-60 minutes later, eat 8-14 ounces (1½-3 cups) raw meat with raw egg(s) and/or 3-10 tablespoons raw butter, raw cream, raw coconut cream, no-salt-added raw cheese with an equal amount of butter or avocado. One or a combination of several raw fats may be eaten at a meal, such as in a sauce.**
- **45-90 minutes later, drink a blended milkshake consisting of 2-4 raw eggs, 3-6 ounces raw milk, 1-4 ounces raw cream and 1-2 tablespoons unheated honey.**
- **At least 1 hour later, drink another 4-12 ounces green vegetable juices.**
- **At least 1 hour later, eat 4-6 ounces fruit with 3-6 ounces of either raw cream, raw coconut cream, raw butter or avocado. You may combine any or all of the above, or you may drink another milkshake without fruit.**
- **At least 1 hour later, drink another 4-12 ounces green vegetable juices.**
- **At least 1 hour later, eat 8-14 ounces (1½-3 cups) raw meat with raw egg(s) and/or 3-10 tablespoons raw butter, raw cream, raw coconut cream, and/or no-salt-added raw cheese with an equal amount of butter or avocado. One or a combination of several raw fats may be eaten at a meal, such as in a sauce.**
- **45-90 minutes later, drink a blended Moisturizing/ Lubrication Formula, page 146.**
- **At least 1 hour later, drink another 4-12 ounces green vegetable juices.**

If you are balanced metabolically, I suggest that you alternate those plans. The recommended daily diets above are intended to cause the weight-gain necessary to remove deep-tissue toxicity.

Weight-loss-Diet Recommendations

❖ Drink 1 cup green vegetable juices.

❖ When very hungry but <u>not in a stupor or angry-hungry,</u> eat 2-3 golfball-sized amounts of meat (any meat that appeals to you) with 1 teaspoon of raw butter, cream or avocado but butter is preferable.

❖ When next very hungry, eat 2 golfball-sized amounts of meat with one teaspoon of raw butter, cream or avocado but butter is preferable.

❖ When next very hungry drink 1 cup green vegetable juices.

❖ When next very hungry, eat 1-2 raw eggs Rocky-style.

❖ When next very hungry, eat 2 golfball-sized amounts of meat with<u>out</u> butter, cream or avocado.

That is one cycle. If the day is not over, start the cycle over. You may eat as many cycles in a day as necessary to avoid eating other food. I suggest that, no matter where you are in a cycle at the end of a day, drink 1 cup of raw milk before a long sleep-period to help relax and calm nerves. If no raw milk is available, drink a blend of 2 ounces raw coconut cream, 4 ounces coconut milk and 1 teaspoon fresh lime juice.

Juice recipe during weight-loss cycle: 1½ tablespoon unheated honey per quart as preservative, ½ small organic lemon or lime with rind per 3 quarts green juice (80% celery, 18% parsley, 2% lemon; percentages are by volume, not weight).

I break the weight-loss diet if I experience lasting detoxification symptoms, such as cold, flu or severe pain. For the recommended diet during bacterial or viral detoxification, see page 147. During detoxification, our bodies need massive nutrients to properly detoxify and heal.

Traveling While Eating The Primal Diet™

While traveling, I always take a minimum of enough meat to last 36 hours. That is usually enough time to get to a store, preferably a healthfood store. For every 14 days of travel, I take 2½ pounds of no-salt-added raw cheeses, 1 quart of unheated honey and 3 pounds of unsalted raw butter. Because I do not drink vegetable juices on trips, I eat many tomatoes, drink coconut milk, chew on celery and expectorate the pulp. Or, I may consume 1 grapefruit per day, or eat other fruit that is low in carbohydrate, such as cherries and berries other than strawberries, with avocado, or butter and cheese. I never eat the cheese without butter. I have a tendency toward constipation when traveling. Usually, it does not bother me. Others have experienced a similar tendency toward constipation while traveling.

When I backpacked in Hawaii and did not have refrigeration, I mixed 5 pounds of butter with 8 ounces (volume) of honey. Only on the 9th day did I detect some fermentation but it was still good and health-giving. My cheese was fine without refrigeration.

Baby Food/Infant Formula
In 1998, a grandmother brought a 12-months-old girl to me. Three months earlier, a Pediatrician had diagnosed the infant with anemia, retardation and oversized liver. The doctor prescribed many supplements, including iron, and specialty baby formulas. After three months on the prescriptions and formulas, the infant showed signs of less strength, more irritability, mental regression, and was unable to sleep restfully.

I placed a golfball-sized amount of finely chopped beef in front of her and let her play with it. Within 15 minutes, she consumed the beef. She took more from the wrapper and ate it. I suggested that the child eat only raw beef, raw milk, unsalted raw butter and a little unheated honey. She improved immediately. Within 2½ months her energy level, mental aptitude and liver were normal. Now, three years later and mainly having continued the diet, she is very advanced physically, mentally, socially and psychically.

For research on infant safety from drinking raw milk and the dangers of drinking formulas, and processed and pasteurized milks, see pages 180-186.

Chapter 13
To Eat Or Not To Eat Spices And Oils?

Spices in small amounts add flavor and excite the taste buds. Eaten too much or too often, spices can cause excessive energy, fatigue, indigestion, gas and constipation. I suggest that we stay attuned to our bodies' changes and the world of spices will be pleasurable. Most spices have been irradiated. Purchase those that are labeled non-irradiated.

As I explained on page 34, pressed oils, such as olive and flax, are used by our bodies as cleansers. They often dry tissue rather than lubricate it. Pressed oils, in many individuals, cause thinning of the mucus that protects the stomach and intestinal linings when oils are eaten too often.

In moderate amounts, mustard increases digestion. If consumed in quantities too high for any individual, raw mustard thins the mucus that protects membranes, and may burn the stomach and intestinal walls. That may result in nervous erratic energy, tense muscles or overall tension. This often causes schizophrenic energy levels as well as exhaustion, sometimes resulting in restless sleep. I consume mustard only to add flavor, and never more than 2 teaspoons per day.

In some individuals, too much onion can cause results similar to that of mustard. The too frequent combination of garlic and onion sometimes creates similar reactions. Consuming too much hot pepper may result in similar side-effects. Too much garlic can cause a similar reaction in some individuals, or create the opposite effects – lethargy and sleepiness – because it may lower blood-pressure too much. Be aware of how these affect you.

Our bodies are always changing and adapting. When using spices, we will gain better health if we are sensitive to our bodies' changing needs. Sometimes an individual may be able to eat spicy food often but then may reach a saturation point and have to stop consuming a particular spice for a period of one day to weeks. Centuries ago, spices were medicine, not condiments. Spices are potent, therapeutic and enjoyable in moderate doses but discomforting when over-consumed or counter-indicated for our bodies' particular requirements. They may cause indigestion accompanied by frequent flatulence.

***

*Let's prepare some health-giving,
tasty food! Bon appetite!*

Chapter 14

Health-Giving Recipes!

Be certain to read all of the instructions on pages 46-50 before making any recipe.

Necessary Equipment
✓ One blender; my preference is an Osterizer.
✓ One juicer; my preference are a Green Star or Green Life because it is a closed-case-crush press. It has the lowest electromagnetic field produced by efficient juicers. I do not use centrifugal juicers because they use air to press the juice from the pulp, oxidizing and damaging up to 30% of the nutrients in the juice.
✓ One 1-quart food processor.
✓ One dozen each of the 12- and 16-ounces regular-sized mouth glass jars; my preference of brand names is *Ball* with enameled lids.
✓ Two dozen each of a 4- and 8-ounces regular-sized mouth glass jars, my preference of brand names is *Ball* with enameled lids. If more than one person lives in the household, many more jars, especially the 8-ounces, will be needed.
✓ Extra enameled regular-sized jar lids to replace rusty lids.
✓ Hand-crank ice cream maker, such as Donvier brand. The hand-crank is best because making ice cream takes approximately 30 minutes. When a motor-driven ice cream maker is used, the high electromagnetic field alters the molecular structure of the food and it is less nutritious, and possibly harmful.

✓ Hand pepper grinder.

Blenderizing The Easy Way

We can blend with many tools, such as a kitchen utensil, food-processor, mixer or blender. I use the word "blenderize" so that there is no mistake that I use a blender. To follow most of the recipes, you will need a blender that accommodates glass jars because most of the recipes utilize small quantities of food. Also, blenderizing in a common blender-bowl sucks oxygen into the bowl and food, oxidizing and damaging approximately 30% of nutrients. It is healthiest and easiest to use the washer, blender-blades and base of a blender that will fit regular-sized-mouth glass jars. As of this writing, all of the blender models made by *Osterizer*, except the Classic model, fit those jars.

Simply remove the base, washer and blades from the blender's bowl and store bowl. Obtain regular-sized-mouth glass jars in the following sizes: 4-ounces, 8-ounces, 12-ounces and 16-ounces.

Sometimes the washer that comes with the blender is too thin and it will not seal properly. The washer should be at least 1/16th-inch thick, but preferably up to 3/32nds-inch thick. Alternative washers of another brand may be obtained at most small appliance and hardware stores. *Do not* use two washers together. Too often one gets caught in the blades.

Place washer on rim of jar, then pass the blades inside jar and rest its plate on top of washer. Ensure that washer and blade-plate are somewhat flush with the jar's rim, and then screw on base firmly. Turn the jar upside down on the blender and start blenderizing.

WARNING! Of the thousands of people who have used the blender blades with glass jars millions of times, I received only one report that the jar broke while it was blending. The gentleman's palm suffered a cut. The washer had gotten caught in the blades and caused the jar to burst. I suspect that the jar was cracked prior to blending. I have had the washer catch on the blades approximately 25 times over 25 five years and the glass never broke. Take your time and be patient. If the washer gets caught in the blades, an unusually deep drone occurs and most often, the ingredients spew from the base of the jar without bursting. Turn off the blender immediately if it sounds strange. Unscrew the base and inspect the washer; is it properly placed? If the washer is too slippery to remain in place, wipe the rim of jar, and rinse and dry the washer before reapplying it to the jar.

Blenderizing Recipes That Include Butter

Blender blades are made of cold metal that will cause butter to chill and stiffen. That often causes the ingredients to freeze-up and not blenderize. When blenderizing a recipe with butter that needs to be melted, it is best to cap the jar with blender washer/blades/base before immersing in mildly hot water. That way, the blades will heat along with the ingredients and blenderizing will be easy.

Making Raw Milk Into Raw Kefir Without A Culture-Additive

Let raw milk stand at room temperature in a dark cupboard. An upper cupboard is preferable because it is warmer. It is ready when the milk becomes thick, usually after two days. Adding 1-2 tablespoons unheated honey help make an enjoyable kefir. If separation of liquid and solids occurs, see making Cottage Cheese, page 59-60.

How To Juice Vegetables And Store Them For 3 Days To Maintain Nutrients

I juice 92 ounces of green vegetable juices at a time for a three-day period. As I juice the vegetables, I pour the juices into a gallon container. After I have juiced 92 ounces (not including foam), I place 3 ounces of juices and 4 ounces of honey in an 8-ounces jar, screw washer/blades/base on jar. I place the jar upside down on the blender and blenderize for 5-10 seconds to thin the honey. I pour the honey/juice mixture into the remaining 89 ounces and gently stir. The honey helps to preserve the juices. Then, I pour the 96 ounces into twelve 8-ounces glass jars. I fill the jars to the top, seal with *Ball*-jar lids and store them in refrigerator. There should be no more than 1 tablespoon of airspace in each jar. My tests showed that refrigerated juices stored that way retained 90 to 93% nutrient value in a 78-hour period.

Making Coconut Cream
1 to 3 Coconuts

Choose a coconut by inspecting its shell. If you find any cracks or dark watermarks, small or large, or black spots, it is probably spoiled. Inspect the three small dark circles grouped together at the top, called eyes. If one of the eyes is open or shrunken, it is spoiled. If the coconut is without any of the above, the odds of having a good coconut are 9 of 10.

Juicing coconuts can seem a chore but the healthful rewards are worth the effort. We will need leather gloves that are not heavily dyed, an ice pick, hammer, oyster knife and a juicer that separates cream from pulp, such as a Green Star juicer.

Poke the coconut eyes until we find the eye that is soft.
Do not puncture it, yet. Puncture one of the hard circles with ice pick and hammer. Then puncture the soft circle with the ice pick. Pour the coconut milk into a glass. Taste the milk. If it is sour, the coconut may be partially or completely spoiled. If the coconut milk (sometimes referred to as coconut water) is good, drink it when thirsty.

Don gloves. Firmly tap coconut shell all around for 2 minutes but not hard enough to crack it yet. That usually loosens the meat from the shell. Now, crack the coconut shell, starting from the bottom, that is, opposite from the three eyes. Hammer the coconut into many pieces. If you find the meat yellow or discolored, it is spoiled or partially spoiled. You can tell where it is spoiled by discoloration on the white meat. Pry the meat from the shell with the oyster knife. If black spots appear on the brown skin, it is spoiled where the spots appear. Separate the non-spoiled meat from the spoiled meat. If it is completely spoiled, begin again with another coconut. Slice good coconut pieces into strips that are approximately 1/4-inch thick x 1/2-inch width and any length. OR! drop the chunks of coconut into a food-processor and grind.

Place the coconut meat slices or ground coconut in a juicer that separates cream from pulp, such as a GreenStar juicer, Champion, or Norwalk. The result is coconut cream that will thicken as hard as butter in refrigeration. Use the pulp to fertilize a garden or lawn. Do not mix coconut milk with the coconut cream unless you intend to drink it within 24 hours; or it will sour. It is best to store coconut cream in many 4-ounces glass jars. Stored in that manner, it will keep for 7 days in refrigeration. If we blenderize 1 tablespoon of lime juice to each 7 ounces of coconut cream, it will preserve for up to 3 weeks. Note: Since making coconut cream requires tools and actions, it is recommended that you juice 3-5 coconuts at a time. Each coconut renders 6-8 ounces of pure cream from a Green Star juicer (do not include the milk from the coconut).

Marinating Meats In Lemon Or Lime Juice

Seafood and Fowl may be marinated in citrus juice. If red meats are marinated in lemon or lime juices or vinegar, often the protein is converted to fuel or solvent rather than for regeneration and cellular reproduction. We obtain more than enough fuel from fat. We should preserve our meat-protein for cellular reproduction. One or two tablespoon of lemon or lime juice or vinegar may be mixed with fat 10 minutes prior to mixing with red meats. Some people say that because fish and fowl look and taste heat-cooked when marinated that they are cooked. That is not true. Like digestive acids in our bodies, citrus juices partially break down the components of food for proper digestion but do not mutilate or destroy the nutrients.

Using Gauze-cloth, Cheesecloth, Or Cheese-pouch For Straining

New material contains bleach and chemical sizing; compounds that are very toxic. Cloth must be thoroughly rinsed in cold and then hot waters, and finally rinsed in warm water with a capful of raw vinegar before use with food. **Do not use soap after the first washing.**

Whipping Raw Cream

When blenderizing cream in a 4-ounces glass jar, always blenderize on low speed. Never use more than 3 ounces of cream in a 4-ounces jar. The cream needs airspace to swell or it will turn into butter. When blenderizing in an 8-ounces jar, blenderize on medium speed. Never use more than 6 ounces of cream in an 8-ounces jar. During blenderizing, when an high pitch from the blender begins, it indicates that the cream is stiff and ready. Turn off the blender.

Making Raw Butter From Raw Cream

Fill an 8-ounces jar with 7 ounces raw cream. Screw on blender washer/blades/base tightly and blenderize for 90 seconds on high speed. Pour off whey.

Ingredients That Are In All Capitalized Letters

A capitalized word indicates that the item itself is a recipe. That recipe must be made first, or made previously.

Quantities And Servings

Most recipes are for 1 serving. To make larger recipes, multiply the appropriate number of servings you need times the amount of each ingredient. If a recipe is for 2 servings and you want to make 4 servings, simply multiply each ingredient by 2.

**** **BABY FOOD** ****

It has been my experience that infants under 1-year old have achieved better health when breast-fed entirely by a mother on a healthy raw animal food diet, especially this Primal Diet. If the mother is not on a healthy diet, I found that the infant gains better health if fed raw milk from a cow or goat rather than mother's milk. The determining factor is, who eats more of a balanced raw food diet, the mother or the animal? Generally, I have observed that children over 9 months of age can easily enjoy the following infant formulas/recipes. In many primitive cultures that do not experience disease, an exclusive raw-milk diet for babies up to 2 years of age has proved perfectly healthful. A few tribes breast feed for up to 4 years and have incredibly healthy children.

Infant Glandular Booster

8 Servings

1   cup organic raw liver
1   cup raw milk
1/4   teaspoon unheated honey

Cut liver into small chunks. Blenderize all ingredients in a 16-ounces jar on high speed for 20-25 seconds. Strain mixture through a strainer or cloth-pouch. Squeeze pouch to speed straining. Use nipple with large hole.

Infant Immune Booster

8 Servings

1   cup organic raw liver
1/2   cup raw milk
2   raw eggs
1/4   teaspoon unheated honey

Cut liver into small chunks. Blenderize all ingredients in a 16-ounces jar on high speed for 20-25 seconds. Strain mixture through a strainer or cloth-pouch. Squeeze pouch to speed straining. Use nipple with large hole.

Infant Milkshake

2 Servings

2	**ounces raw milk**
2	**ounces raw cream**
1	**raw egg**
1/4	**teaspoon unheated honey**

Blenderize all ingredients together in an 8-ounces jar on medium speed for 5 seconds. No straining is necessary.

Infant Nervous System Booster

8 Servings

1	**ounce fresh ocean wild-caught raw fish**
3	**tablespoons raw cream**
1/4	**cup fresh organic liver**
2	**ounces raw milk**
1	**raw egg**
1/2	**teaspoon unheated honey**

Cut liver and fish into small chunks. Blenderize ingredients in an 8-ounces jar on high speed for 20-25 seconds. Strain mixture through a strainer or cloth-pouch. Squeeze pouch to speed straining. Use nipple with large hole.

**** **BEVERAGES** ****

Green Vegetable Juices
These juices provide more than the necessary vitamin-, enzyme- and mineral-supplementation that is necessary, they help the functions described in their title. Read pages 30-31, regarding the addition of clay to vegetable juices.

Helps Regulate Body Salts, Remove Toxic Salts, And Increase Oxygen Absorption

12 Servings

5	bunches fresh celery stalks (with leaves if not wilted)
5	bunches fresh parsley, curly or Italian
3-4	ounces unheated honey (help to preserve the juices as well as sweeten them)

Read page 47, regarding proper storage of juices to maintain nutrient-value.)

Helps Remove Impactions (Plaque)
From Arteries And Intestines,
Regulate Body Salts, And Increase Oxygen Absorption

12 Servings

4	bunches fresh celery stalks (with leaves if not wilted)
3	bunches fresh parsley, curly or Italian
3	medium carrots
3	ounces unheated honey (help to preserve the juices as well as sweeten them)
1/2	-inch circular slice pineapple. dice

Blenderize diced pineapple into an 8-ounces jar on medium speed for 10 seconds. Follow the rest of instructions for juicing and proper storage of juices to maintain nutrient-value on page 47.

Helps Eliminate Toxicity From Liver, Other Glands,
Decrease Lymphatic Congestion,
Regulate Body Salts, And Increase Oxygen Absorption

12 Servings

4	bunches fresh celery stalks (with leaves if not wilted)
3	bunches fresh parsley, curly or Italian
1	lemon, juice rind and all
1	bunch fresh cilantro
2	medium raw zucchini, crookneck or sunburst squash
1	medium cucumber
3	ounces unheated honey (help to preserve the juices as well as sweeten them)
12	tablespoons coconut cream.

Read page 47, regarding proper storage of juices to maintain nutrient-value.)
Immediately before drinking this juice formula, eat 1 tablespoon coconut cream, unsalted raw butter or raw cream.

Helps Remove & Eliminate Mercury
And Other Heavy Metals,
Regulate Body Salts, And Increase Oxygen Absorption

12 Servings

3	bunches fresh celery stalks (with leaves if not wilted)
3	bunches fresh parsley, curly or Italian
3	bunches fresh cilantro
4	medium raw zucchini, crookneck or sunburst squash (occasionally cucumber)
3	ounces unheated honey (helps to preserve the juices as well as sweetens them)
12	tablespoons raw cream, or
12	tablespoons coconut cream, or unsalted raw butter.

Often, the body pulls heavy metals from its cells and tissues with the nutrients in this juice. Fats must be present with the juice to ensure that detoxified metals do not cause harm and restore in the body. Therefore, immediately before drinking this juice formula, eat 1 tablespoon coconut cream or butter, or drink a little juice and put 1 tablespoons raw cream into the juice and stir.

Read page 47, regarding proper storage of juices to maintain nutrient-value.

Milkshake
(Soothes nerves.)

1 Serving

1 to 3	raw eggs
3 to 6	ounces raw milk
2 to 4	ounces raw cream
1 to 2	tablespoons unheated honey

Blenderize in an appropriately sized jar on medium speed for 5-10 seconds.

Coffee Substitute

(Most often, any mixture of green vegetable juices is the best substitute for coffee. Green vegetable juices fill the digestive tract and blood with energy producing vitamins, enzymes and minerals, and usually increase appetite for healthy food.)

1 Serving

4	ounces natural mineral water
2	tablespoons unheated honey
2	tablespoons lemon or lime juice
1	tablespoon raw apple cider vinegar
2	tablespoons raw cream

Blenderize all ingredients, except cream, in an 8-ounces jar on medium speed for 5-10 seconds. Pour in cream and stir. If you would like it warm, cap and immerse in mildly hot water for 5 minutes.

Banana Smoothie

Fruity milkshakes make some people more emotional, sensitive, irritable and/or sleepy. If you experience those symptoms, you would probably do better by drinking milkshakes.

1 Serving

2 to 3	raw eggs
1/3	banana
3	ounces raw milk
1	ounce raw cream
1	pinch freshly ground nutmeg
1	tablespoon unheated honey

Blend all ingredients together in an 8- or 12-ounces jar on medium speed for 10 seconds.

Orange Smoothie

Fruity milkshakes make some people more emotional, sensitive, irritable and/or sleepy. If you experience those symptoms, you would probably do better by drinking milkshakes.

1 Serving

2 to 3	raw eggs
1	peeled and seeded orange
2	ounces raw cream
1	teaspoon unheated honey, (optional)

Blenderize all ingredients together in an 8-ounces jar on high speed for 10 seconds.

Raspberry Smoothie

Fruity milkshakes make some people more emotional, sensitive, irritable and/or sleepy. If you experience those symptoms, you would probably do better by drinking milkshakes.

1 Serving

2 to 3	raw eggs
4	ounces raspberries
1	ounce raw milk
2	ounces raw cream
1	teaspoon unheated honey

Blenderize all ingredients together in an 8- or 12-ounces jar on medium speed for 10 seconds.

**** COTTAGE CHEESE ****

Caraway Cottage Cheese

4 Servings

1	quart raw milk
3	ounces raw cream
1 1/2	tablespoons caraway seeds

Pour milk into a wide-mouthed quart jar, add caraway seeds and let stand in a dark high cupboard until the liquid completely separates from the solids (2-4 days). Pour into a cheese-making cloth-pouch, or make a pouch from gauze-cloth or several layers of cheesecloth. Hang and let strain until milk solids are firm but not too dry. (Use the whey to pickle, or in place of raw vinegar to prepare sauces and spices, or mix whey with 5 parts water and feed to indoor or outdoor plants.)

Put firm cheese in bowl and gently stir in 3 ounces raw cream.

Sour Cottage Cheese

4 Servings

1   quart raw milk
3   ounces raw cream

Pour milk into a wide-mouthed quart jar and let stand in a dark high cupboard until the liquid completely separates from the solids (2-4 days). Pour into a cheese-making cloth-pouch, or make a pouch from gauze-cloth or several layers of cheesecloth. Hang and let strain until milk solids are firm but not too dry. (Use the whey to pickle, or in place of raw vinegar to prepare sauces and spices, or mix whey with 5 parts water and feed to indoor or outdoor plants.)

Put firm cheese in bowl and gently stir in 3 ounces raw cream.

Sweet Cottage Cheese

4 Servings

1   quart raw milk
3   ounces raw cream

Pour milk into a wide-mouthed quart jar and let stand in refrigeration until cream separates to the top. Skim the cream off of milk, place cream in an 8-ounces jar, cap and place cream in refrigerator. Let milk stand in quart jar in a dark high cupboard until the liquid completely separates from the solids (2-4 days).

Pour into cheese-making cloth pouch, or make pouch from gauze-cloth or several layers of cheesecloth. Hang and let strain until milk solids are firm but not dry. (Use the whey to pickle, or in place of raw vinegar to prepare sauces and spices, or mix whey with 5 parts water and feed to indoor or outdoor plants.)

Put firm cheese in bowl and stir in separated cream and an additional 3 ounces raw cream.

**** MEAT MEALS ****

White meats are fowl, fish, seafood, pork, rabbit, squirrel and other small animals. **Red meats** are beef, lamb, bison, venison, and other large animals.

Preparing Meat Dishes

There are seven basic preparations for meat: Whole, sliced, diced, chopped, ground, pâté, and liquefied. Each preparation has a distinct flavor. Liquefied meats are usually for invalids and infants. However, liquefying glands is an easy way for anyone to eat glands. Pâté the meats in a food processor, then, using a blender, blenderize them with an equal amount of raw milk, and a little honey if desired, in a glass jar until they are liquid.

I have observed that most people prefer the carpaccio-style of meat preparation, that is, meat sliced very thinly, especially tough meats. Most butchers and restaurants freeze the meat in order to slice it very thinly. Frozen meat does not give much healing or cellular-reproductive support to the body. Frozen meat produces more byproducts and toxins than fresh meat. It is better to slice it thinly by using the slicing plate in a food processor. Other people like meats thick and juicy at room temperature, or ground. Taste is in the palate of the eater.

The flavors of sauces change according to whether we blenderize, chop, crush, grate, marbleize, whip, stir or fold ingredients. Sauces produce distinct flavors according to how we combine them with meats. We may stir or fold in, marbleize, pour over, sprinkle, mash into, marinate, or blend sauces with meats. Using one sauce to blend with meat and topping it with another sauce, gives more options and flavors. As we make sauces with suggested alternatives, we will understand infinite possibilities. I present one or two alternatives per meat dish; see pages 87-113. Adventure and explore flavors as our tastebuds change.

Even though I have hundreds of sauce-recipes, usually I eat meats plain. When I spice meats, usually it is a time when I am repulsed by or bored with plain meats. If I do not eat meats daily, after a day or two I do not feel or function as well. Sauces help me eat meats at those times. I found that force-feeding myself provides the nutrients necessary to live a healthier life in our toxic world. I encourage my clients to do so, too, especially those who are anorexic.

Meat Sauces

All of the following sauces may be used with red or white meats: beef, lamb, venison, bison, pork, fowl, fish and seafood.

Asian Spicy Meat Sauce

2 Servings

1	raw egg
7	tablespoons raw cream
1	tablespoon finely grated fresh ginger root
1/2	teaspoon unheated honey
1	tablespoon MUSTARD

Ingredients should be room temperature except mustard. Blenderize all ingredients, except cream, together in a 4-ounces jar on medium speed for 10 seconds. Blenderize cream in an 4-ounces jar on low speed until cream is stiff. Gently fold blended mixture into whipped cream.

Barbecue Sauce

2 Servings

1	tomato, medium
1/4 to 1/2	fresh hot pepper, such as jalapeno
4	tablespoons stone-pressed olive oil
1	teaspoon raw unpasteurized apple cider vinegar
1	teaspoon finely chopped fresh basil
1	teaspoon finely chopped fresh thyme
1/8	teaspoon minced fresh garlic, (optional)
1	teaspoon diced fresh red onion

If a thicker sauce is desired, slice a deep and wide cut in tomato. Over a bowl , gently squeeze tomato to remove juice and seeds. Drink tomato juice when thirsty. Blenderize all ingredients, except onion, together in an 8-ounces jar for 7 seconds. Stir onion into sauce, or sprinkle over sauce after sauce is poured over meat.

Béchamel Sauce

1 Serving

2	tablespoons unsalted raw sunflower seeds
2	tablespoons raw milk
3	tablespoons unsalted raw butter
1	pinch freshly grated nutmeg
1	teaspoon chopped fresh thyme
1/4	teaspoon chopped fresh red onion
1	pinch ground white pepper

All ingredients must be room temperature. Warm the milk, butter, nutmeg, onion and pepper together in a 4-ounces jar immersed in a bowl of mildly hot water for 5 minutes. When butter is liquid, blenderize together for 10 seconds on low speed. In another 4-ounces jar, blenderize seeds on medium speed for 5 seconds. Add seed flour to sauce and blenderize for 10 seconds on low speed.

Bordelaise Sauce

1 Serving

2	tablespoons bone marrow
2	tablespoons raw cream
1	tablespoon unsalted raw butter
1	teaspoon chopped fresh leeks
1	teaspoon grated fresh turnips
1	tablespoon grated no-salt-added raw cheese

Scoop the marrow from bone. Warm all ingredients, except cheese, in a 4-ounces jar, capped with blender washer/blades/base, immersed in bowl of mildly hot water for 5 minutes. Blenderize together on low speed for 10 seconds. Stir in grated cheese.

Bordelaise Sauce, Two

1 Serving

4	tablespoons bone marrow
2	sugar-cubed-sized cubes fresh pineapple
1/2	teaspoon chopped shallots
1/4	teaspoon chopped bay leaves
1/8	teaspoon chopped thyme
1	pinch freshly ground mixed peppercorns
1/2	teaspoon fresh lemon juice
1	sliced fresh mushroom

Scoop the marrow from bone. Warm all ingredients, except mushroom and shallot, together in a 4-ounces jar, capped with blender washer/blades/base, in bowl of mildly hot water for 5 minutes. Blenderize on low speed for 10 seconds.

Add sauce to meat, arrange sliced mushrooms and top by sprinkling with shallot.

Caesar Meat-Dressing

1 Serving

2	tablespoons walnut halves
1	egg, or 4 tablespoons stone-pressed olive oil
2	teaspoons fresh lemon juice
1	tablespoon raw cream
1	teaspoon unheated honey
1/2	teaspoon freshly chopped thyme
1	slice fresh garlic

Blend walnuts in an 8-ounces jar for 5 seconds on medium speed. Add all other ingredients and blend on low speed for 10 seconds.

Cheesy Spiced Paste

4 Servings

1	cup SOUR COTTAGE CHEESE
2	ounces SPICE PASTE

Mash and stir together until thoroughly mixed. Will keep in refrigeration for 2 weeks.

Creamy Cheese Pepper Sauce

1 Serving

2	tablespoons grated no-salt-added raw cheese
2	tablespoons raw cream
1/2	medium tomato
1	teaspoon MUSTARD
1/3	jalapeno
1/4	hot red pepper
1	teaspoon finely chopped fresh bay leaves, (optional)

If a thicker sauce is desired, slice a deep and wide cut in tomato. Over a bowl, gently squeeze tomato to remove juice and seeds. Drink tomato juice when thirsty. Place all ingredients in an 8-ounces jar and blenderize for 5-10 seconds.

Egg/Cheese Basil Sauce

1 Serving

2	tablespoons unsalted raw butter, or raw cream, or raw milk
1	egg
4	tablespoons grated no-salt-added raw Monterey cheese
2	tablespoons finely chopped fresh basil leaves
1	diced tomato
1	teaspoon PICKLED PEPPERS (PIMENTOS), (optional)

Blenderize egg, 1 tablespoon basil and cheese together in an 8-ounces jar on medium speed until smooth.

Slice beef thinly lengthwise, and slice again to make small rectangles. Place meat and diced tomato in a decorative pattern on plate. Pour sauce over meat. Sprinkle with pimentos and remaining chopped basil.

French Mayonnaise

3 Servings

2	eggs
2	teaspoons MUSTARD
1/2	teaspoon fresh lemon juice
6	tablespoons chilled unsalted raw butter
6	tablespoons stone-pressed olive oil
2	pinches ground white pepper

Blend all ingredients together in a 12-ounces jar on medium speed for 15-20 seconds.

Garlic Butter

2 Servings

6	tablespoons raw unsalted butter
1	(or more) thin slice of a single section of garlic clove
1/8	teaspoon unheated honey, (optional)

Place all ingredients together in a 4-ounces jar, capped with blender washer/blades/base, immersed in mildly hot water until melted. Blenderize on medium speed for 5 seconds.

Hollandaise Meat Sauce

2 Servings

4	tablespoons raw unsalted butter
1/2	teaspoon MUSTARD
1	tablespoon grated horseradish
1/2	medium tomato
1	teaspoon unheated honey
2	tablespoons stone-pressed olive oil

All ingredients should be room temperature. If a thicker sauce is desired, slice a deep and wide cut in tomato. Over a bowl, gently squeeze tomato to remove juice and seeds. Drink tomato juice when thirsty. Blenderize all ingredients together in an 8-ounces jar on medium speed for 5 seconds.

Hollandaise Meat Sauce, Two

1 Serving

3	tablespoons unsalted raw butter
1	raw egg
1/2	teaspoon fresh lemon juice
1/4 to 1/2 fresh hot pepper	

Butter should be room temperature, firm but not cold. Blend all ingredients together in a 4-ounces jar on low speed for 5 seconds.

Horseradish Sauce

8 Servings

6	tablespoons grated fresh horseradish
3	tablespoons raw cream
3	tablespoons raw milk
1/2	teaspoon unheated honey
1/2	teaspoon fresh raw lime juice, (optional)

Blenderize all ingredients together in an 8-ounces jar on medium speed for 10 seconds. It will keep for 2 months in refrigeration.

Horseradish Sauce, Two

8 Servings

7	tablespoons grated fresh horseradish
5	tablespoons raw milk, or whey, or 1 tablespoon raw apple cider vinegar and 4 tablespoons whey
1	tablespoon unheated honey
1	tablespoon fresh lime juice

Blenderize all ingredients together in an 8-ounces jar on medium speed for 10 seconds. It will keep for 2 months in refrigeration.

Italian Sauce

2 Servings

5	ounces stone-pressed olive oil
1	tablespoon finely chopped rosemary
1	tablespoon finely chopped basil
1/4	garlic clove, pressed, (optional)

Stir all ingredients together in an 8-ounces jar for 1 minute. Cap and let stand in cupboard for at least 3 days. Do not refrigerate at any time.

If you would like to flavor a bottle of olive oil, triple the quantities of rosemary, basil and garlic, add to bottle of oil and let stand for at least 3 days.

Ketchup

2 Servings

1	tomato
1	tablespoon unsalted raw butter
1	tablespoon stone-pressed olive oil
1	teaspoon unheated honey
1/2	teaspoon raw apple cider vinegar
1	teaspoon fresh red onion
1	slice fresh garlic
1	pinch freshly ground mixed peppercorns
1	teaspoon fresh fish eggs, (makes for salty taste), (optional)
1	teaspoon MUSTARD, or SPICE PASTE

Slice a deep and wide cut in tomato. Over a bowl, gently squeeze tomato to remove juice and seeds. Drink tomato juice when thirsty.

Place tomato and all ingredients in an 8-ounces jar and blenderize on medium speed for 10 seconds. If ingredients stick to bottom and do not blend properly, remove from blender and shake jar until ingredients unsettles at blades, replace on blender and resume blenderizing.

Mayonnaise

2 Servings

4	tablespoons unsalted raw butter
1	raw fertile egg
1	tablespoon fresh raw lemon juice
1/2	teaspoon unheated honey
1/2	teaspoon raw unpasteurized apple cider vinegar
4	tablespoons stone-pressed olive oil

All ingredients should be room temperature. Blenderize all ingredients together in an 8-ounces jar on medium speed until smooth.

Mexican Sour Cream Sauce

6 Servings

1	slice minced fresh garlic
2	tablespoons chopped fresh red onion
1	tomato
2	tablespoons chopped fresh cilantro
1	cup SOUR CREAM

Slice a deep and wide cut in tomato. Gently squeeze tomato in hand over a bowl to remove juice and seeds. Drink tomato juice when thirsty.

Chop tomato and stir/fold all ingredients together. It will keep in refrigeration for 3 weeks.

Mornay Sauce

1 Serving

2	ounces BECHAMEL SAUCE
1	tablespoon raw cream
1	raw egg
2	pinches ground white pepper
2	tablespoons grated no-salt-added raw cheese

Blenderize egg, cream, and pepper together in a 4-ounces jar on low speed for 10 seconds. Add Béchamel Sauce and cheese, and stir/marbleize. Spoon over slivered raw meat.

Mousseleine Sauce

1 Serving

2	ounces HOLLANDAISE MEAT SAUCE, TWO
2	ounces raw cream

Blenderize cream in a 4-ounces jar on low speed until it is stiff. Swirl/marbleize Hollandaise sauce into whipped cream.

Mushroom Cream Cheese Sauce

1 Serving

1	large mushroom
2	tablespoons raw cream
3	tablespoons no-salt-added raw cheddar cheese
1	raw egg

Chop mushroom and set aside. Cut cheese into small chunks. Blenderize all ingredients, except half of the chopped mushroom, together in a 4-ounces jar on low speed for 10 seconds. Stir in remaining chopped mushroom.

Mushroom Cream Sauce

1 Serving

1	large mushroom
1	tablespoon unsalted raw butter
3	tablespoons raw cream
2	tablespoons raw milk
2	teaspoons diced fresh red onion, (optional)

Chop mushroom. Blenderize all ingredients, except half of the chopped mushroom and onion, together in an 8-ounces jar on medium speed for 15 seconds. Stir in remaining chopped mushrooms and onion.

Mustard

10 Servings

4	tablespoons whole yellow mustard seeds
4	tablespoons whole brown mustard seeds
3	ounces whey or natural mineral water
3	tablespoons raw unpasteurized apple cider vinegar
1 to 2	tablespoons unheated honey

Place mustard seeds, vinegar and whey together in an 8-ounces jar. Pour in enough whey, or water, to fill jar. Cap and let it stand at room temperature in cupboard for 24 hours. Add honey and blenderize on medium speed for 15 seconds. It will keep in refrigeration for several months.

Mustard, Two

10 Servings

3	tablespoons whole yellow mustard seeds
3	tablespoons whole brown mustard seeds
2	tablespoons unheated honey
3	tablespoons raw apple cider vinegar
4	ounces whey or natural mineral water
2	pinches freshly grated nutmeg
1	teaspoon chopped fresh watercress

Place mustard seeds, vinegar and whey together in an 8-ounces jar. Pour in enough whey, or water, to fill jar. Cap and let stand at room temperature in cupboard for 24 hours. Add honey, nutmeg and watercress. Blenderize on medium speed for 15 seconds. It will keep in refrigeration for several months.

Mustard Butter

1 Serving

1 to 2   tablespoon MUSTARD
3 to 4   tablespoons unsalted raw butter

Vigorously stir or marbleize mustard into soft butter.

Nut And Spice Sauce

1 Serving

2   ounces pine nuts
2   tablespoons stone-pressed olive oil
2   tablespoons unsalted raw butter
1 to 3   teaspoons unheated honey
1/2   teaspoon raw apple cider vinegar
1/2   slice garlic, (optional)
1   tablespoon fresh red onion, chopped, (optional)

Blenderize nuts into flour in a 4-ounces jar on medium speed. Warm butter and oil in an 8-ounces jar, capped with blender washer/blades/base, immersed in a bowl of mildly hot water for 5 minutes. Add nut flour, honey, vinegar and garlic and blenderize on low speed. Stir in onion.

Pepita Gravy

1 Serving

2	ounces pumpkin seeds
2	ounces meat-fat trimmings or unsalted raw butter
2	tablespoons raw cream
1	teaspoon unheated honey, (optional)

Warm meat-fat or butter with cream in a 4-ounces jar, capped with blender washer/blades/base, immersed in bowl of mildly hot water for 5 minutes.

Blenderize pumpkin seeds into flour in a 4-ounces jar on medium speed. Add fat or butter, cream and honey, and blenderize on low speed, for 15-20 seconds, until it won't blend or it is smooth.

Sour Cream

8 Servings

24	ounces raw cream

Pour cream into a quart jar, loosely screw on lid, and let stand in the refrigerator for 1-3 months. Scoop out as you want it. When you reach the bottom, you will find whey. Use the whey in recipes, or dilute with 5x more water than whey and feed to plants.

Sour Cream Quick

1 Serving

4	tablespoons raw cream
3	tablespoons grated no-salt-added cheese

Blenderize cream and cheese together in a 4-ounces jar on low speed until thick and firm (10-15 seconds).

South African Frikkadel Glaze

1 Serving

2	ounces pecan halves
1	egg
2-4	tablespoon chopped fresh red onion
1	pinch freshly grated nutmeg
1	pinch freshly ground coriander seeds
1	pinch freshly ground mixed peppercorns
2	ounces meat-fat trimmings or unsalted raw butter
1	tablespoon stone-pressed olive oil
2	tablespoons unheated honey

Blenderize pecans in an 8-ounces jar until they are flour. Add egg, nutmeg, coriander, peppercorns, fat or butter, oil and honey, and blenderize on medium speed for 15 seconds. Add sauce to meat and top with chopped red onion.

Spice Paste

8 Servings

2	whole cardamon seeds
1	teaspoon coriander seeds
1	teaspoon whole allspice
1/2	cinnamon stick
1	shallot
1	tablespoon fresh tarragon leaves
1/4	teaspoon white pepper
1	teaspoon mixed peppercorns
1	teaspoon fenugreek seeds
2	pistils of saffron
1	fresh hot pepper
5	ounces stone-pressed olive oil

If you enjoy a less hot paste, remove seeds from fresh hot pepper. Blenderize all ingredients, except fresh hot pepper and shallot, together in an 8-ounces jar on medium speed for 5 seconds and on high speed for another 5 seconds.

Add and blenderize all ingredients together in an 8-ounces jar on medium speed for 20 seconds. Cap and let stand in cupboard for 24 hours, then use or refrigerate. Paste will keep in refrigeration for approximate 3 months.

Spiced Butter or Oil

2 Servings

6	ounces unsalted raw butter, or olive oil, or flax oil
1	slice garlic clove
1	teaspoon freshly grated ginger root
1	pinch turmeric
1	pinch freshly ground cardamon seed
1	pinch freshly ground cloves
1	pinch nutmeg, freshly ground
1	teaspoon fresh red onion, (optional)

Warm butter in an 8-ounces jar, capped with blender washer/blades/base, immersed in a bowl of mildly hot water for 5 minutes. Blenderize all ingredients together on medium speed for 15 seconds.

If using oil, there is no need to immerse in hot water before blenderizing.

ALTERNATIVE: Stir in onion after blenderizing all other ingredients together.

Spicy African Paste

4 Servings

2	tomatoes
6	tablespoons stone-pressed olive oil
3	tablespoons unsalted raw butter
1	whole cardamon seed
1/4	teaspoon coriander seeds
1/4	teaspoon grated fresh ginger root
1/4	teaspoon fenugreek seeds
1	whole clove
1/4	inch cinnamon stick
1/4	teaspoon whole allspice
1	slice fresh garlic clove
1/2	teaspoon fresh red onion
1	pinch paprika
3	whole mixed peppercorns
1	pinch grated nutmeg
1/4	fresh hot red pepper
1	tablespoon unheated honey

Blenderize cardamon, coriander, fenugreek, clove, cinnamon, allspice and peppercorns together in a 4-ounces jar until they are flour.

If a thicker sauce is desired, slice a deep and wide cut in tomato. Over a bowl, gently squeeze tomato to remove juice and seeds. Drink tomato juice when thirsty. Blenderize all ingredients together in a 12- or 16-ounces jar for 15 seconds. Let stand for at least 10 hours. Sauce will keep in refrigeration for at least 1 month.

Spicy Thai Sauce

1 Serving

2	ounces walnut halves
1/4	stalk celery
1/2	teaspoon fresh ginger root
3	tablespoons coconut cream
1/2	tablespoon unheated honey
1	tablespoon chopped Thai basil, or mint leaves, (optional)
½-4	tablespoons fresh hot peppers (authentic Thais make it so hot their noses perspire while they eat).

Blenderize celery and ginger together and strain out pulp. Warm coconut cream in a 4-ounces jar, capped with blender washer/blades/base, immersed in a bowl of mildly hot water for 5 minutes.

Blenderize walnuts in an 8-ounces jar until they are flour. Add juices, honey and coconut cream and blenderize all ingredients together on medium speed for 10 seconds. If ingredients stick to bottom while blending, remove from blender and shake loose, then resume blending.

ALTERNATIVE 1: Rather than blenderize basil into sauce, cover meat with sauce and top with sprinkled basil.

ALTERNATIVE 2: Stir all ingredients together for 1 minute rather than blenderizing.

Tango Meat Sauce

1 Serving

3	tablespoons room-temperature soft raw unsalted butter
1	teaspoon grated horseradish, or HORSERADISH recipe
1/2	tomato
1	teaspoon unheated honey
2	tablespoons olive oil

If a thicker sauce is desired, slice a deep and wide cut in tomato. Over a bowl, gently squeeze tomato to remove juice and seeds. Drink tomato juice when thirsty.

Blenderize all ingredients together in an 8-ounces jar on medium speed for 10 seconds.

ALTERNATIVE 1: Blenderize all ingredients, except mustard, together on medium speed for 10 seconds. Stir-marbleize mustard into sauce.

ALTERNATIVE 2: Blenderize all ingredients, except tomato, together in a 4-ounces jar on medium speed for 10 seconds. Dice tomato and fold into sauce.

Tartar Coconut Cream Sauce

1 Serving

1	tablespoon finely chopped fresh dill weed
4	tablespoons coconut cream
1	tablespoon fresh lemon juice
1	tablespoon fresh lime juice
1	tablespoon chopped PICKLE

All ingredients must be room temperature except dill. Finely chop dill. Blenderize all ingredients, except pickles together, in a 4-ounces jar on low speed for 10 seconds. Add and stir in pickles. Eat with meat, or marinate at room temperature for 1 hour to enhance flavors.

Tartar Sauce

2 Servings

2	tablespoons lemon juice
1	teaspoon unheated honey
6	tablespoons raw unsalted butter
1	raw egg
2	tablespoons fresh dill weed
1	tablespoon finely diced fresh red onion, (optional)
1	tablespoon chopped PICKLE

All ingredients must be room temperature except dill. Finely chop dill. Blenderize all ingredients, except onion and pickle, together in an 8-ounces jar on medium speed for 10 seconds. Stir in chopped onion and pickle. Pour on meat. Eat, or marinate at room temperature for 4 hours.

Thousand Island Meat-Dressing

1 Serving

2	ounces cherry tomatoes
1	tablespoon stone-pressed olive oil
1	raw egg
1	tablespoon unsalted raw butter
1/2	tablespoon fresh red onion
1	slice fresh garlic

Blenderize all ingredients in an 8-ounces jar on medium speed for 10 seconds.

Thousand Island Meat-Dressing, Two

4 Servings

2	tablespoons fresh lemon juice
1 1/2	teaspoons unheated honey
3/4	cup cherry tomatoes
1	teaspoon vinegar
2	tablespoons olive oil
1/2	-inch cube of no-salt-added raw Monterey cheese
1	teaspoon fresh red onion, (optional)
1	slice fresh garlic, (optional)

Cut cheese into thin slices. Blenderize all ingredients together in a 12-ounces jar on high speed for 10-15 seconds. This dressing will keep in refrigeration for several weeks in closed jar.

Tomato Cream Cheese Sauce

1 Serving

2	tablespoons raw cream
1/2	diced tomato
1	teaspoon fresh lemon juice
1	-inch cube of no-salt-added raw cheese
2	tablespoons grated no-salt-added raw cheese

If a thicker sauce is desired, slice a deep and wide cut in tomato. Over a bowl, gently squeeze tomato to remove juice and seeds. Drink tomato juice when thirsty. Blenderize all ingredients, except grated cheese, together in a 4-ounces jar on low speed for 10 seconds. Pour over meat and top with sprinkled grated cheese.

Tomato Sauce

1 Serving

1/2	tomato
4	tablespoons raw unsalted butter, (or stone-pressed olive oil)
1/2	-inch cube of no-salt-added raw cheese
1	slice fresh garlic

1/2 to 1 tablespoon chopped fresh red onion
Favorite fresh herbs to your taste , (optional)

All ingredients should be room temperature. If a thicker sauce is desired, slice a deep and wide cut in tomato. Over a bowl, gently squeeze tomato to remove juice and seeds. Drink tomato juice when thirsty. Warm butter in an 8-ounces jar, capped with blender washer/blades/base, immersed in bowl of warm water until butter melts. Add rest of ingredients to jar and blenderize on medium speed for 10 seconds.

Wasabe

4 Servings

6	tablespoons grated fresh wasabe or horseradish
2	ounces natural mineral water, or whey
1	teaspoon unheated honey
1	teaspoon fresh lemon juice
1/3	avocado
1/4	teaspoon raw apple cider vinegar

Blenderize all together in an 8-ounces jar on medium speed for 15 seconds.

White Pepper Sauce

1 Serving

1	raw egg
2	tablespoons unsalted raw butter
2	tablespoons raw cream
1	pinch grated nutmeg
2	pinches ground white pepper

Blenderize all ingredients together in a 4-ounces jar on low speed for 10-15 seconds.

Red Meat Meals

Beef, lamb, venison, buffalo, pork and wild meat. Any meat, including fowl, fish or seafood may be substituted for the specified meat in the recipe.

Himalayan Meat

1 Serving

5 to 8   ounces raw meat (beef, lamb, fowl, seafood)
2 to 3   ounces CHEESY SPICED PASTE

Chop meat into bite-sized pieces.
Spread paste on plate and cover with chopped meat.

ALTERNATIVE: Cut meat into strips and spread paste on strips.

African Lamb

1 Serving

1/4	teaspoon raw apple cider vinegar
1/2	teaspoon unheated honey
1/4	teaspoon grated fresh ginger root
1/2	freshly ground clove
5	tablespoons unsalted raw butter
3	seedless raisins
1	slice crushed fresh garlic
1	pinch freshly ground peppercorns
5 to 8	ounces lamb

Warm all ingredients, except ginger and meat, in a 4-ounces jar, cap with blender washer/blades/base, immersed in bowl of mildly hot water. When butter has completely melted, blenderize on medium speed for 10 seconds. Add and stir in ginger.

Prepare lamb as you wish and add or cover with sauce.

ALTERNATIVE 1: Replace butter with stone-pressed olive oil.

ALTERNATIVE 2: Reduce unsalted raw butter to 2 1/2 tablespoons and add 2 1/2 tablespoons stone-pressed olive oil.

Beef Pâté

1 Serving

4	tablespoons pumpkin seeds
4	tablespoons unsalted raw butter
1	slice fresh garlic
5 to 8	ounces ground beef
1	teaspoon diced red onions
1	egg

Blenderize seeds in an 8-ounces jar on medium speed for 5 seconds. Warm butter and garlic in a 4-ounces jar, capped with blender washer/blades/base, immersed in a bowl of mildly hot water for 5 minutes. Blenderize butter and garlic on low speed for 5 seconds. Pour butter/garlic into seed flour in an 8-ounces jar, stir and blenderize on medium speed for 5 seconds. Place meat and all ingredients into food processor and blend until they are paste.

Beef Stroganoff

1 Serving

5 to 8	ounces chopped beef
1	slice minced garlic
3	chopped mushrooms
2	chopped chives
5	tablespoons SOUR CREAM or SOUR CREAM QUICK

Stir garlic and sour cream together. Lay bed of mushrooms, cover with meat, top with sour cream and sprinkle with chives.

Carpaccio (pronounced carpachio)

1 Serving

5	tablespoons stone-pressed olive oil
2	tablespoons grated no-salt-added raw cheese
1	tablespoon finely chopped fresh bay leaves
1	tablespoon finely chopped fresh basil leaves
1	tablespoon chopped fresh parsley
1	slice minced or crushed fresh garlic, (optional)
1	teaspoon chopped fresh red onion, (optional)
5 to 8	ounces meat (beef, lamb, fowl, seafood)
1	mushroom

Vigorously stir olive oil, bay, basil, onion and garlic together for 1 minute.

Slice meat into thin luncheon meat-sized slices in food processor with slicing plate. In a covered bowl at room-temperature, marinate meat slices in sauce for 1 to 3 hours.

Spread meat and sauce on plate and sprinkle with cheese and top with parsley.

Ethiopian Kitfo

1 Serving

1 to 2	**tablespoon SPICE PASTE**
1	**teaspoon red onions**
1/2	**teaspoon fresh hot pepper**
1/2	**teaspoon freshly grated fresh ginger root**
1	**pinch freshly ground cardamon seed**
1	**tablespoon lemon juice**
1/4	**red, yellow and/or green bell pepper**
5 to 8	**ounces fresh beef**

Mash paste, pepper, ginger, cardamon and lemon together in a cup.

Cut meat into chunks and place in food processor. Add all ingredients and blend all together for 10 seconds.

Lamb Shanks

1 Serving

5 to 8	ounces lamb shanks
2	tablespoons unsalted raw butter
1	teaspoon bone marrow
3	tablespoons stone-pressed olive oil
1 to 2	tablespoons grated raw unsalted Monterey cheese
1	teaspoon chopped fresh basil, (optional)
1	teaspoon chopped fresh bay leaves, (optional)
1	tablespoon chopped fresh parsley
1	spear asparagus
1	teaspoon chopped red onions, (optional)
1	slice minced fresh garlic, (optional)

Scoop marrow from shank bone. Warm butter, oil, basil and/or bay leaves and garlic together in a 4-ounces jar, capped with blender washer/blades/base, immersed in bowl of mildly hot water for 5 minutes. When butter has melted, blenderize ingredients for 5 seconds at medium speed.

Slice lamb into strips. Dice asparagus. In a covered bowl at room temperature, marinate lamb strips and asparagus in sauce for 1-3 hours. Spread marinated ingredients on plate and top with cheese, onion and parsley.

Liver Pâté

1 Serving

5 to 8   **ounces organic raw liver**
1 to 3   **tablespoons red onions, (optional)**

Cut liver into small chunks. Put liver and onion in food processor and blend together for 20-30 seconds.

Liver Pâté, Two

1 Serving

2 to 4   **tablespoons raw sunflower seeds**
5 to 8   **ounces organic raw liver**
1 to 3   **tablespoons red onions, (optional)**

Blenderize sunflower seeds in a 4-ounces jar on medium speed for 10 seconds. Cut liver into small chunks. Put all ingredients in food processor and blend together for 20-30 seconds.

Meat au Gratin

1 Serving

4	tablespoons unsalted raw butter, (may substitute stone-pressed olive oil)
1	slice fresh garlic
1/4	red bell pepper
1 1/2	-inch cube no-salt-added raw cheddar cheese
5 to 8	ounces raw meat (beef, lamb, fowl, seafood)

Grate a portion of room-temperature cheese and set aside. Slice remaining cheese thinly. Warm cheese slices, garlic and room-temperature butter in a 4-ounces jar, capped with blender washer/blades/base, immersed in bowl of mildly hot water for 5 minutes. When butter is completely melted, blenderize ingredients until smooth.

Cut 1/8 bell pepper into circular slices. Chop remaining 1/8 bell pepper. Slice meat thinly lengthwise. Arrange meat on plate in overlapping circular pattern. Pour sauce over meat. Cover with slices of bell pepper like spokes of a wheel. Sprinkle grated cheese on top. Finish by sprinkling with chopped bell pepper.

Nuts Over Meat

1 Serving

4 to 5	ounces NUT BUTTER
5 to 8	ounces raw meat (beef, lamb, fowl, seafood)
1/4	quarter of a zucchini or cucumber, or combination

Make nut butter of choice.

Slice zucchini and/or cucumber circularly and place on plate in circle. Slice meat into thin strips and place inside squash circle. Pour nut butter over meat.

Steak Tartare

1 Serving

5 to 8	ounces raw sirloin steak, or New York steak
2	tablespoons red onions
1 to 3	tablespoons unsalted raw butter
1	raw egg
1	teaspoon raw MUSTARD
2	pinches freshly ground caraway seeds
2	pinches freshly ground mixed peppercorns
1/2	teaspoon unheated honey, (optional)
1	teaspoon horseradish, (optional)
1	sprig parsley or cilantro

Cut steak into cubes. Blend meat and all ingredients together in food processor for 5-15 seconds, depending on the desired consistency.

White Meat Meals - Fowl

Chicken, turkey, duck and wild birds.   Any meat may be substituted for the specified meat in the recipe.

Cajun Chicken

1 Serving

2	tablespoons refrigerated unsalted raw butter
1	tablespoon refrigerated raw cream
1	chilled raw egg (keep refrigerated for 2 hours)
1	pinch freshly grated nutmeg
1	pinch fresh ground mixed peppercorns
5 to 8	ounces raw chicken
1/2	diced tomato

Blenderize egg, nutmeg, pepper, chilled butter and cream in a 4-ounces jar on low speed for 4-6 seconds.

Dice chicken. Fold sauce with chicken and top with diced tomato.

Cheesy Chicken

1 Serving

5   tablespoons stone-pressed olive oil
1   tablespoon fresh lemon juice
1   -inch cube sliced no-salt-added raw cheese
1/4 to 1 fresh hot pepper
1   teaspoon fresh red onion, (optional)

Blenderize all ingredients, except chicken, together in a 4-ounces jar on medium speed for 10 seconds. Slice chicken into narrow strips, baste and marinate for 20-60 minutes.

ALTERNATIVE: Instead of blenderizing onion, dice and gently stir into sauce before basting and marinating chicken.

Chicken Salad

1 Serving

5 to 8   ounces raw chicken
1   tablespoon diced cucumbers
1   tablespoon chopped summer squash
1   tablespoon PICKLED PEPPERS (PIMENTOS)
3   tablespoons MAYONNAISE

Place chicken in food processor, blend for 5-7 seconds and place in bowl. Add all other ingredients and gently fold into ground chicken.

Chicken/Beef Mustard

1 Serving

2 to 3   ounces ground or diced raw chicken
3 to 5   ounces diced beef
2   tablespoons grated no-salt-added raw Monterey cheese
1   serving MUSTARD BUTTER

Fold meats and mustard/butter together and top with cheese.

French Chicken

1 Serving

2   tablespoons SOUR CREAM or SOUR CREAM QUICK
1/2   diced tomato
1/2   teaspoon finely chopped bay leaves
1/2   teaspoon finely chopped thyme
1/2   teaspoon freshly ground mixed peppercorns
1/4   crushed fresh garlic clove
1/2   teaspoon chopped parsley
5 to 8   ounces raw chicken

Place chicken in food processor and blend for 10 seconds. Spread a thick layer of chicken on plate. Gently stir garlic and sour cream together. Spread layer of sour cream over meat. Spoon tomato over sour cream and sprinkle with ground peppercorns, bay, thyme and parsley, in that order.

Macaroni & Cheese-Tasting Chicken

1 Serving

6   ounces chopped or ground raw chicken
3   tablespoons SOUR CREAM
1   egg
1   red hot pepper
3   tablespoons grated no-salt-added raw cheese

Blenderize egg, pepper, cheese and sour cream together in an 8-ounces jar on medium speed for 10 seconds. Fold sauce into chicken.

ALTERNATIVE: On a plate, form chicken into a plateau, indent and fill with sauce.

Orange-Glazed Duck

1 Serving

3   tablespoons soft unsalted raw butter
1   pinch black pepper, (optional)
1   section fresh orange
1   tablespoon unheated honey
1/4   teaspoon raw apple cider vinegar
1/2   teaspoon lemon juice
1   fresh mint leaf
5 to 8   ounces raw duck

Blenderize all ingredients, except duck and mint, in a 4-ounces jar on high speed for 5 seconds.

Chop duck into small pieces. Cover with orange glaze. Marinate for 2 hours

Finely chop mint leaf and sprinkle over glaze.

Parmesan Chicken

1 Serving

6	**ounces raw chicken, dice**
4	**walnut halves**
2	**tablespoons stone-pressed olive oil**
1	**tablespoon fresh lemon juice**
2	**tablespoons raw cream**
1	**tablespoon finely chopped oregano**
1	**slice minced garlic clove**

Blenderize walnuts into flour in a 4-ounces jar on high speed for 5 seconds. Add all ingredients, except chicken, and blenderize on low speed for 15 seconds. Spread over chicken. Eat immediately or marinate for 45 minutes.

Salsa Chicken

1 Serving

1	tomato
1	fresh hot pepper
2	tablespoons fresh lime juice
1/2	teaspoon vinegar
5 to 8	ounces skinned, boned, diced chicken breast
1/4	diced red bell pepper
1/4	stalk diced celery
1	slice avocado, or
1	raw egg
1	tablespoon diced red onions
1	sprig cilantro, (optional)

Slice a deep and wide cut in tomato. Over a bowl, gently squeeze tomato to remove juice and seeds. Drink tomato juice when thirsty. Blenderize tomato, pepper, vinegar, and lime juice together in an 8-ounces jar on medium speed for 5-10 seconds. Pour sauce over chicken in a bowl, fold together and marinate for 45 minutes. Top with other ingredients and eat from bowl.

ALTERNATIVE: Spoon chicken on to plate, cover with sauce and spread remaining ingredients on top.

Sexy Chicken

1 Serving

5 to 8   ounces skinned, boned, diced chicken breasts
1   raw egg
4 to 5   ounces NUT BUTTER made with peanuts
1   inch section chopped celery stalk
1   tablespoon chopped fresh arugula leaves

Gently whip raw egg, peanut butter, celery and arugala together in a small bowl. Fold chicken into whipped mixture. Spoon spiced chicken on to plate. Pour remaining sauce in bowl over chicken.

ALTERNATIVE: Gently whip raw egg, peanut butter and celery together in a small bowl. Spread chicken on plate, cover with sauce and top with arugala.

Tahitian Chicken

1 Serving

3   ounces COCONUT CREAM
1/2 to 1 diced tomato
2   tablespoons fresh lemon juice
2   tablespoons fresh lime juice
5 to 8   ounces fresh raw chicken

Stir coconut cream and lime juice together, and let stand for 10 minutes.

Dice meat. Place chicken, lemon juice and tomato in a bowl and fold gently together. Top with coconut/lime sauce. Eat immediately or let marinate 2 hours before topping with coconut/lime sauce.

Turkey Pâté

1 Serving

5 to 8	**ounces turkey**
1 to 2	**raw eggs**
1 to 2	**tablespoons MUSTARD, and/or HORSERADISH**
1	**tablespoon diced red onions**
1/2	**diced tomato**

Place turkey in food processor and blend for 20 seconds. Mash turkey down into food processor and add egg(s) and mustard and/or horseradish and blend for 10 seconds more. Put into bowl or on plate and cover with tomato and onion.

ALTERNATIVE: When adding egg and mustard, or egg and horseradish to food processor, add tomato and onion. Blend for 10 seconds.

POWER DRINKS

Liver Booster

1 Serving

4 to 8	**ounces organic raw liver**
4 to 8	**ounces raw milk**
1	**tablespoon unheated honey, (optional)**

Cut liver into small chunks. Blenderize all ingredients together in a 12- or16-ounces jar on high speed for 20 seconds.

Liver Booster, Two

1 Serving

4 to 8   ounces organic raw liver
4 to 8   ounces raw milk
1 to 2   tablespoons red onions, (optional)

Cut liver into small chunks. Blenderize all ingredients together in a 12- or16-ounces jar on high speed for 20 seconds.

The Power Drink

1 Serving

2   tablespoons organic raw liver
1   tablespoon organic raw thyroid gland
1   tablespoon organic raw testis or ovary
2   tablespoons organic raw lung
1   tablespoons organic raw brain
1   tablespoon organic adrenal gland
4   ounces raw milk
1 to 2   tablespoons red onions

Blenderize all ingredients together in a 12-ounces jar on high speed for 20 seconds.

Seafood/Fish Sauces

Island Fish Sauce

1 Serving

1	ounce banana or pineapple
1	tablespoon unsalted butter
1	raw egg
1/4	teaspoon unheated honey, (optional)
1	drop organic vanilla extract, (optional)

Blenderize all ingredients together in a 4-ounces jar on high speed for 10 seconds.

Polynesian Ginger Sauce

1 Serving

1	tablespoon coarsely grated fresh ginger root
2	tablespoons fresh lemon juice
1	tablespoon unheated honey
2 to 3	tablespoons unsalted raw butter, room temperature

Vigorously stir butter and all other ingredients together.

Spicy African Paste for Fish

4 Servings

2	tomatoes
6	tablespoons flax oil
3	tablespoons unsalted raw butter
1	whole cardamon seed
1/4	teaspoon coriander seeds
1/4	teaspoon grated fresh ginger root
1/4	teaspoon fenugreek seeds
1	whole clove
1/4	inch cinnamon stick
1/4	teaspoon whole allspice
1	slice fresh garlic clove
1/2	teaspoon red onions
1	pinch paprika
3	whole mixed peppercorns
1	pinch grated nutmeg
1/4	fresh hot red pepper
1	tablespoon unheated honey

Blenderize cardamon, coriander, fenugreek, clove, cinnamon, allspice and peppercorns together in a 4-ounces jar on high speed until they are flour.

If a thicker sauce is desired, slice a deep and wide cut in tomato. Over a bowl, gently squeeze tomato to remove juice and seeds. Drink tomato juice when thirsty. Blenderize all ingredients together in a 12- or 16-ounces jar on medium speed for 15 seconds. Let stand for at least 10 hours. Sauce will keep in refrigeration for at least 1 month.

White Meat Meals - Seafood/Fish

Any fish, seafood or fowl may be substituted for the specified meat in the recipe.

Ceviche

1 Serving

5 to 8	ounces fresh ocean wild-caught raw fish
3 to 4	ounces fresh lemon or lime juice
1/2 to 1	diced fresh tomato
4 to 6	tablespoons flax oil, or stone-pressed olive oil
1	tablespoon chopped fresh cilantro
1	tablespoon chopped red onion, (optional)
1	slice minced fresh garlic, (optional)

Dice fish and marinate in lemon or lime juice for 20 minutes to 24 hours in a jar or bowl.

Stir oil, onion and garlic together for 1 minute. Pour off lemon or lime juice from fish. Pour oil mixture over fish. Top with diced tomato.

Escolar Fresca

1 Serving

5 to 8	ounces Escolar fish
1/2	diced tomato
2	tablespoons fresh lime or lemon juice
1	tablespoon diced apples
1	teaspoon diced red onion, (optional)
1	teaspoon unheated honey, (optional)

If using honey, mix lime or lemon juice with honey until honey is dissolved. Stir tomato, apple and onion together and spoon over fish. Marinate for 10-40 minutes.

Hot Buttered Salmon

1 Serving

5 to 8   ounces fresh ocean wild-caught raw salmon
3   tablespoons lemon or lime juice
1/8 to 1/2 hot pepper
3   tablespoons raw unsalted butter
2   tablespoons grated no-salt-added raw cheese

Warm lemon and lime juices, hot pepper and soft butter together in a 4-ounces jar, capped with blender washer/blades/base, immersed in a bowl of mildly hot water for 5 minutes. Blenderize on medium speed for 10 seconds. Pour mixture over salmon and top with grated cheese.

Oyster Sauce & Pasta

1 Serving

1   serving PASTA SUBSTITUTE
3   oysters
2   mushrooms
2   tablespoons raw unsalted butter
1 1/2   -inch cube raw unsalted Monterey or Muenster cheese
1   slice red or white onion
2   tablespoons fresh sweet red pepper, (optional)

Make PASTA SUBSTITUTE (see recipe). Blenderize 1 1/2 oysters, 1 mushroom, butter, 1/2 of the cheese, 1/2 of the onion and 1/2 of the red pepper together in an 4-ounces jar on medium speed for 10 seconds. Dice remaining oysters, mushrooms and onion. Fold diced ingredients together with sauce and pour over PASTA. Grate remaining cheese. Top dish with grated cheese.

ALTERNATIVE: Follow recipe above but do not blenderize onion in sauce. Chop onion and fold into sauce.

Oysters Over Cheese

1 Serving

5	**fresh oysters**
2	**mushrooms**
5	**tablespoons unsalted raw butter**
6	**tablespoons grated no-salt-added raw cheese**
1	**teaspoon chopped red onions**
1 to 2	**circular slice(s) fresh sweet red peppers, (optional)**

Blenderize 1 1/2 oysters and butter in a 4-ounces jar on high speed for 10 seconds.

In a food processor, chop with pulse-action the sweet pepper, mushrooms and remaining oysters. In a serving bowl, fold all ingredients, except cheese, together.

Sprinkle a bed of cheese evenly over plate. Spoon oyster/pepper/mushroom mixture evenly over cheese. Top with oyster/butter sauce.

Salmon with Lemon And Parsley

1 Serving

5 to 8   ounces salmon, chopped, bite-sized pieces
6 to 9   tablespoons fresh lemon or lime juice
1/2   cup finely chopped fresh parsley

Marinate fish in juice for at least 20 minutes at room temperature. Place fish on plate and sprinkle with parsley.

Shrimp Passion

1 Serving

5 to 8   ounces fresh shrimp
1   teaspoon grated fresh ginger root
1   teaspoon chopped red onions, (optional)
1/4 to 1/2 finely chopped fresh hot pepper
1/3   partially ripe papaya
1   tablespoon chopped fresh parsley

Sprinkle ginger over papaya and mash together until saucy, or chop papaya and blenderize with ginger in a 4-ounces jar on high speed for 5-10 seconds.

Stir in pepper and onion. Spoon over shrimp and top by sprinkling with parsley.

Spiced Salmon

1 Serving

5 to 8	**ounces fresh ocean wild-caught raw salmon**
1	**tablespoon slivered shallots**
2	**tablespoons unsalted raw butter**
1	**sliced mushroom**
1	**tablespoon chopped fresh dill**
1	**egg**
1	**tablespoon fresh lemon juice**
1/4 to 1/2	**chopped fresh hot pepper**

Blenderize egg, chilled butter, dill, and lemon juice together in a 4-ounces jar on high speed for 5 seconds.

Cut salmon into strips and arrange in circular pattern on plate. Cover with blended mixture. Arrange shallot slivers on top and sprinkling with chopped hot pepper.

Spiced Sashimi

1 Serving

1	**tablespoon grated fresh ginger root**
1	**teaspoon WASABE, or HORSERADISH**
3	**tablespoons flax oil**
1	**tablespoon very soft unsalted raw butter**
1/2	**teaspoon unheated honey, (optional)**
5 to 8	**ounces fresh ocean wild-caught raw fish**

Vigorously stir all ingredients together, or blenderize in a 4-ounces jar on low speed for 5 seconds. Spoon over fish.

Swordfish Sashimi

1 Serving

5 to 8	ounces fresh Swordfish
4	tablespoons fresh lemon or lime juice
1	fresh hot pepper (like jalapeno)
2	ounces stone-pressed olive oil
	small assortment of herbs or lettuce

Grate and finely chop pepper. Stir juice, olive oil and pepper together for 1 minute. Slice swordfish into strips. Arrange fish in a pattern on plate. Pour oil/juice/pepper mixture over fish.

Tahitian Fish

1 Serving

3	ounces COCONUT CREAM
1/2 to 1 diced tomato	
3 to 4	tablespoons fresh lime juice
5 to 8	ounces fresh ocean wild-caught raw fish

Stir coconut cream and lime juice together and let stand for 10 minutes.

Dice meat. Place fish and tomato in a bowl. Pour coconut/lime sauce over fish and tomato and fold gently together. Eat immediately or let marinate for up to 8 hours.

ALTERNATIVE: Substitute 1/3 cup pineapple for tomato.

Thai Ceviche

1 Serving

5 to 8   ounces fresh ocean wild-caught raw fish
4 to 6   tablespoons fresh lemon or lime juice
2 to 4   tablespoons flax oil, or stone-pressed olive oil
1 to 2   tablespoons unsalted raw butter
1   tablespoon chopped fresh mint, (optional)
2   tablespoons chopped PICKLED GINGER

Dice fish and marinate in lemon or lime juice for 20 minutes or up to 24 hours. Pour off juice.

Stir oil, soft butter and ginger together for 1 minute and pour over fish. Top with chopped mint.

ALTERNATIVE: Use all oil, or all butter, or varying amounts of oil and butter.

**** SOUP ****

Chicken & Tomato Soup

1 Serving

3 to 5   ounces chopped raw chicken
1 1/2 to 2 tomatoes
2   drops organic vanilla extract
1 1/2   teaspoons raw apple cider vinegar
1   tablespoon unheated honey
2   tablespoons stone-pressed olive oil

Place all ingredients into food processor and blend for 5 seconds. Pour into bowl.

Chicken Soup

1 Serving

5 to 8	**ounces raw chicken**
1	**tablespoon chopped watercress**
2	**tablespoons unsalted raw butter**
1	**slice red onion, or shallot, or coarsely chopped chives**
3	**ounces raw milk**
2	**tablespoons stone-pressed olive oil**
1	**pinch freshly ground mixed peppercorns**

Warm butter, oil, milk and watercress in an 8-ounces jar, capped tightly and immerse jar in a bowl of mildly hot water until butter completely melts.

Place all ingredients, including chicken, in food processor and blend for 10-15 seconds.

If you would like warm soup, place soup in a 16-ounces jar, cap and immersed in bowl of mildly hot water for 10 minutes.

Cream of Chicken Soup

1 Serving

5 to 8	**ounces raw chicken**
1	**egg**
1/4	**teaspoon raw apple cider vinegar**
1	**teaspoon unheated honey, (optional)**
1	**tablespoon stone-pressed olive oil**
1	**tablespoon unsalted raw butter**
4	**tablespoons raw milk**
2	**tablespoons raw cream**
1	**tablespoon SPICE PASTE**
1	**tablespoon raw sunflower seeds**

Add all ingredients to food processor and blend for 5-10 seconds. Pour into bowl.

Grandma's Tomato Soup

1 Serving

1 1/2 to 2 tomatoes
2   drops organic vanilla extract
1 1/2   teaspoons raw apple cider vinegar
1   tablespoon unheated honey
2   tablespoons stone-pressed olive oil

Place all ingredients into food processor and blend for 5 seconds. Pour into bowl.

Lentil Soup

1 Serving

2   tablespoons whole sprouting lentils, do not sprout
3   ounces natural mineral water
1   tablespoon sunflower seeds
1   ounce raw milk
2   ounces raw cream
1   tablespoon unsalted raw butter
1   raw egg
1   slice fresh garlic
1   teaspoon unheated honey

Place lentils in a 4-ounces jar and fill jar to top with water. Place in cupboard and let stand for 24 hours. Drain off water and blenderize for 4 seconds.

Blenderize sunflower seeds in another 4-ounces jar on high speed for 5 seconds. Blenderize all ingredients, except 1/2 of the ground lentils, into a 12-ounces jar on medium speed for 20-30 seconds. Stir in remaining ground lentils.

If you prefer warm soup, put a tight lid on jar and immerse in mildly hot water for 10 minutes.

Split Pea Soup

1 Serving

2	tablespoons whole sprouting peas, do not sprout
3	ounces natural mineral water
1	tablespoon sunflower seeds
1	ounce raw milk
2	ounces raw cream
1	tablespoon unsalted raw butter
1	raw egg
1	slice fresh garlic
1	teaspoon unheated honey

Place peas in a 4-ounces jar and fill jar to top with water.
Place in cupboard and let stand for 24 hours. Drain off water and
blenderize for 4 seconds.

Blenderize sunflower seeds in another 4-ounces jar on high
speed until they are flour. Blenderize all ingredients in a 12-
ounces jar and blenderize on medium speed for 15-20 seconds.

If you prefer warm soup, put a tight lid on jar and immerse in
mildly hot water for 10 minutes.

**** RAW STARCH ****

Breads, crackers, pasta, cakes, cookies and products made from beans, potatoes, yams and grains should not be eaten because acrylamides and Advanced Glycation End products (glycotoxins) store in a healthy body at a rate of 70%, and in an unhealthy body at a rate of 90%. Cooked carbohydrates are for those who cannot manage their tempers, and should only be eaten at times when eating raw fowl and/or seafood, and/or raw-nut formula, and abstaining from sweet fruits, do not reduce hyperactivity and temper-tantrums.

Nut Butter/Nut Formula

1 to 2 Servings

2 to 4   ounces raw pecans or walnuts, pine or hazel nuts, sunflower or pumpkin seeds, or peanuts
4 to 8   tablespoons unsalted raw butter
1 to 2   raw egg
1½ to 2 tablespoon unheated honey

Blenderize nuts in an 8- or 12-ounces jar on high speed until they are flour. Add remaining ingredients and stir. Blenderize on medium speed for 20-25 seconds, until smooth.

ALTERNATIVE: Substitute coconut cream for butter.

Pasta Substitute

1 Serving

3   ounces raw sunflower seeds
1/2   teaspoon unheated honey
1   raw egg
1   tablespoon unsalted raw butter

Blenderize sunflower seeds in an 8-ounces jar on high speed for 5-10 seconds. Add butter, honey and egg, and stir together. Blenderize on medium speed for 15 seconds.

Spread mixture evenly on plate and let stand in refrigerator for 2 hours. Cover with any sauce.

Reminiscent of Mexican Chips

1 Serving

3   tablespoons soft unsalted raw butter
1/4 to 1/2 fresh hot pepper
1/4   tomato
2   tablespoons grated Monterey Jack cheese
1   slice fresh garlic, (optional)
1   tablespoon red onions, (optional)
1   serving PASTA SUBSTITUTE

Blenderize butter, tomato, hot pepper, garlic and/or onion together in an 8-ounces jar on medium speed for 10 seconds. Add cheese and blenderize on medium speed for 15-20 seconds, until smooth and warm to the touch. Pour over Pasta Substitute and eat before it gets soggy. Eat with a serving of meat.

Reminiscent of Refried Beans

1 Serving

2	ounces raw pumpkin seeds
1	ounce raw sunflower seeds
3	tablespoons raw unsalted butter
1/4	teaspoon unheated honey
1	raw egg
1	slice fresh garlic

Blenderize pumpkin and sunflower seeds in an 8-ounces jar on high speed until they are flour. Add butter, honey, garlic and egg and blenderize on medium speed for 15-20 seconds. Place in cupboard and let stand for 2 hours.

Top with a sauce and eat with a serving of meat.

**** SWEET MEALS ****

Cheesecake

10 Servings

3/4   **pound no-salt-added raw cheddar cheese**
1   **pound unsalted raw butter**
1   **cup raw walnut halves**
3   **tablespoons unheated honey**
1   **drop organic vanilla extract**

TOPPING, (optional)
1 1/3 **cups raw cream**
1   **tablespoon unheated honey**

Let cheese and butter stand at room temperature to warm for 4 hours before making cheesecake.

Slice cheese into 1/8-inch slices. Into each of two 16-ounces jars, warm half of the cheese, half of the butter and 1 tablespoon honey immersed in a bowl of mildly hot water while making the Crust.

Crust: In a food processor (not blender), place nuts, two tablespoons butter and 1 tablespoon honey. Blend ingredients until they become a large ball.

Butter bottom and sides of an 8- or 9-inch pie plate. Evenly spread nut mixture and press on to bottom of pie plate. Chill in freezer while making Filling.

Filling: When butter is nearly liquid, blenderize both jars of butter/cheese/honey mixture on high speed for 60-90 seconds until ingredients are smooth, not grainy. Do not let it get too hot while blending. Pour both jars of Filling into chilled piecrust and refrigerate for several hours. (If making a Topping, place back in freezer while making Topping.)

ALTERNATIVE TOPPING 1:   Blenderize 5 ounces cream and 1 teaspoon honey in an 8-ounces jar on low speed until it is fluffy and stiff. Repeat with remaining 5 ounces cream and 2 teaspoons honey in another 8-ounces jar. Remove pie from freezer and top with whipped cream. Let stand in refrigeration for 8 hours. The flavors blend better when it stands for 20 hours.

ALTERNATIVE TOPPING 2:   Choose fruit with low carbohydrate, such as cherries, berries and/or unripe fruit. Remove seeds or stones. Chop fruit, if necessary, and blenderize 1 cup fruit and 1 tablespoon honey in a 12-ounces jar on medium speed for 10 seconds. Spread over chilled cheesecake.

ALTERNATIVE TOPPING 3:   Remove stones from 4 dates. Chop dates. Blenderize chopped dates and 1 cup fruit(s) in a 12-ounces jar on high speed for 15 seconds. Spread over chilled cheesecake.

Cheesecake, Miniature

2 Servings

3	ounces no-salt-added raw cheddar cheese
3 1/2	ounces unsalted raw butter
2	ounces raw walnut halves
2	teaspoons unheated honey
1	drop organic vanilla extract

TOPPING, if desired

3	ounces raw cream
1	teaspoon unheated honey

Let cheese and butter stand at room temperature to warm for 4 hours before making cheesecake.

Slice cheese into 1/8-inch slices. Warm cheese, butter and 1 teaspoon honey in an 8-ounces jar, capped and immersed in a bowl of mildly hot water while making the Crust.

Crust: Blenderize nuts, 1 teaspoon butter and 1 teaspoon honey together in a 4-ounces jar on high speed using pulse-action for 5 seconds.

Butter bottom and sides of 4-inch glass or ceramic pie-dish. Evenly spread nut mixture and press on to bottom of pie plate. Chill in freezer while making Filling.

Filling: Blenderize butter/cheese/honey mixture on high speed for 30-40 seconds until ingredients are smooth, not grainy; do not let it get too hot while blending. Pour into chilled piecrust and place in refrigerator for several hours. (If making a Topping, place back in freezer while making Topping.)

ALTERNATIVE TOPPING 1: Blenderize 3 ounces cream and 1 teaspoon honey in an 8-ounces jar on low speed until it is fluffy and stiff. Remove pie from freezer and top with whipped cream. Let stand in refrigeration for 8 hours. The flavors blend better when it stands for 20 hours.

ALTERNATIVE TOPPING 2: Choose fruit with low carbohydrate, such as cherries, berries and/or unripe fruit. Remove seeds or stones. Chop fruit, if necessary, and blenderize 3 ounces fruit and honey in a 4-ounces jar on medium speed for 5 seconds. Spread over chilled cheesecake.

ALTERNATIVE TOPPING 3: Remove stones from 1 date. Chop date. Blenderize chopped date and 3 ounces fruit(s) in a 4-ounces jar on high speed for 10-15 seconds. Spread over chilled cheesecake.

Coconut Cream & Fruit

1 Serving

4	ounces COCONUT CREAM
1/8	peeled and seeded small papaya
1/8	-inch circular slice fresh pineapple
1	teaspoon unheated honey, (optional)

If pineapple is not organic, wash outside of pineapple with brush and lukewarm water. Slice pineapple circularly. Cut away rind and discard. To retain juice in pineapple, slice and dice pineapple with sawing motion. Fold diced fruit into coconut cream, or top diced fruit with coconut cream, or top coconut cream with diced fruit.

ALTERNATIVE: Use 2 ounces each of other fruits, such as berries and peach, or nectarine and peach, or pear and grapes.

Custard

1 Serving

1/3	**papaya, remove seeds and peel**
1	**raw egg**
2	**tablespoons raw unsalted butter**
1	**tablespoon unheated honey**

Blenderize all ingredients together in an 8-ounces jar on low speed for 10 seconds. Immediately pour into serving bowl before it thickens, or let it thicken in jar and eat from jar.

Custard Aphrodisiac

1 Serving

1	**egg**
1/3	**diced avocado**
1/2	**diced orange**
1	**tablespoon unheated honey**
4	**ounces papaya or mango**
1	**teaspoon lime, (optional)**
4	**tablespoons unsalted raw butter**

Blenderize butter, papaya or mango, honey, egg, and lime juice together in an 8-ounces jar on high speed for 10 seconds. Immediately pour into bowl and stir in diced avocado and orange before it thickens. Let stand for 3-5 minutes.

Fudge Parfait

or

Mint Fudge Parfait

2 Servings

5	ounces raw cream
3	tablespoons raw milk
1	raw egg
3	tablespoons peeled and seeded fresh papaya
2	teaspoons unheated honey
2	-inch square PECAN FUDGE

Premake PECAN FUDGE recipe

Blenderize 2 ounces cream, milk, egg, papaya and honey in an 8-ounces jar on medium speed for 5 seconds. Pour into a serving bowl, place in freezer and let sit for 10-16 hours, or use ice cream maker.

Cut fudge of choice into thin layers and place one layer in dessert glass. Spoon a layer of ice cream on top. Repeat the two layers.

Blenderize 3 ounces cream in a 4-ounces jar on low speed until cream is stiff. Top fudge/ice cream layers with whipped cream.

ALTERNATIVE: Chop mint leaves until you have 1 tablespoon. Blenderize 3 ounces cream and chopped mint in a 4-ounces jar on low speed until mixture is stiff. Top fudge/ice cream layers with mint whipped cream.

Gingerbread Balls

1 Serving

3	tablespoons unsalted raw butter
1	tablespoon unheated honey
1	teaspoon grated fresh ginger root
1	tablespoon raw carob powder
2 1/2	ounces raw walnut or pecan halves, pine or hazel nuts, or sunflower seeds

Warm butter and ginger in a 4-ounces jar, capped and immersed in a bowl of mildly hot water.

Blenderize nuts in an 8-ounces jar on high speed until they are flour (or pulse-blend to make it chunky). When butter melts, add honey and blenderize for 5 seconds. Add nuts and carob powder and stir for 60 seconds. Put on plate and let stand for 2 hours until it firms. Form into balls. To harden it more, refrigerate for 30 minutes.

ALTERNATIVE 1: Make it chewier by using honeycomb.

ALTERNATIVE 2: Stir in 1 teaspoon soft fresh bee pollen.

ALTERNATIVE 3: Finely grate coconut meat and roll balls in grated coconut.

Mint Chocolate Substitute

2 Servings

7	tablespoons soft unsalted raw butter
1	raw egg
3	tablespoons finely chopped fresh mint leaves
2	tablespoons unheated honey
1 1/2	tablespoons raw carob powder
2	drops organic vanilla extract

Blenderize all ingredients together in an 8-ounces jar on medium speed for 30-40 seconds. Refrigerate to harden for 2 hours. (To preserve the nutrients in eggs, it is best not to refrigerate for more than 4 hours.)

Pecan Fudge

1 Serving

2	ounces pecan halves
4	tablespoons unsalted raw butter
1	raw egg
3	tablespoons unheated honey
2	tablespoons raw carob powder
1	drop organic vanilla extract

Blenderize pecans in an 8-ounces jar on high speed until they are flour. Place the rest of ingredients in jar, stir, and blenderize on medium speed until smooth. Place in a small bowl and refrigerate to harden for 2 hours. (To preserve the nutrients in eggs, it is best not to refrigerate for more than 4 hours.)

ATERNATIVE 1:   To make it chunky, place all ingredients, except 1 ounce pecans, in an 8-ounces jar and blend until smooth. Crush 1 ounce pecans into bits and stir into mixture. Place in a small bowl and refrigerate to harden for 2 hours.

ALTERNATIVE 2:   Substitute walnuts, pine or hazelnuts for pecans.

South African Chipolata

1 Serving

2	sections tangerines
1/2	tablespoon grated fresh ginger root, or **PICKLED GINGER**
1	tablespoon unheated honey
1	egg
1/4	papaya, peeled and seeded
2	tablespoons unsalted raw butter
5	tablespoons raw cream
1	pinch nutmeg

Blenderize all ingredients, except cream and nutmeg, together in an 8-ounces jar on high speed for 10 seconds. Pour into serving bowl immediately before it solidifies into custard.

Blenderize cream in a 4-ounces jar on low speed until it is stiff. Top custard with whipped cream and grate nutmeg on top.

Whipped Cream Ambrosia

1 Serving

4	**ounces raw cream**
7	**fresh berries**
1/4	**cup diced fresh pineapple**
1	**teaspoon unheated honey, (optional)**

Blenderize cream and honey in an 8-ounces jar on low speed until it is stiff. Place fruit in bowl and top with whipped cream.

ALTERNATIVE: Use other fruits, such as berries and peach, or nectarine and peach, or pear and grapes.

Whipped Cream Tropical

1 Serving

4   **ounces raw cream**
1/8   **peeled and seeded small papaya**
1/8-inch circular slice fresh pineapple
1   **teaspoon unheated honey**

If pineapple is not organic, wash outside of pineapple with brush and lukewarm water. Slice pineapple circularly. Cut away rind and discard. To retain juice in pineapple, slice and dice pineapple with sawing motion. Blenderize cream and honey in a 4-ounces jar on low speed until it is stiff. Fold diced fruit into whipped cream, or top diced fruit with whipped cream, or top whipped cream with diced fruit.

Ice Cream

Berry Good Ice Cream

1 Serving

1	egg
4	tablespoons raw cream
3	tablespoons raw milk
3	tablespoons fresh berries, such as blueberries, raspberries, boysenberries and blackberries
1	tablespoon unheated honey

Blenderize all ingredients together in a 12-ounces jar on medium speed for 10 seconds. Pour into ice cream maker and churn until firm.

French Vanilla Ice Cream

2 Servings

1	egg
4	tablespoons raw cream
4	tablespoons raw milk
3	tablespoons fresh papaya
1	tablespoon unsalted raw butter
1	tablespoon unheated honey
2	drops organic vanilla extract

Blenderize all ingredients together in a 12-ounces jar on medium speed for 10 seconds. Pour into ice cream maker and churn until firm.

Gingerbread Ice Cream

1 Serving

1	egg
4	tablespoons raw cream
4	tablespoons raw milk
1	tablespoon raw carob powder
1	tablespoon unheated honey
1 to 2	teaspoons grated fresh ginger root

Blenderize all ingredients together in a 12-ounces jar on medium speed for 10 seconds. Pour into ice cream maker and churn until firm.

Lime Ice Cream

1 Serving

1	egg
4	tablespoons raw cream
4	tablespoons raw milk
2	tablespoons fresh lime juice
1	tablespoon unheated honey

Blenderize all ingredients together in a 12-ounces jar on medium speed for 10 seconds. Pour into ice cream maker and churn until firm.

Pineapple Ice Cream

1 Serving

1	egg
4	tablespoons raw cream
3	tablespoons raw milk
1 1/2	ounces fresh pineapple
1	tablespoon unheated honey

Blenderize all ingredients together in a 12-ounces jar on medium speed for 10 seconds. Pour into ice cream maker and churn until firm.

Cream Sickles

These cream sickles satisfy without causing manic behavior, as most common sweets do. Refrigerating egg is an exception for this recipe.)

Mango Creamsickles

4 Servings

1	egg
4	tablespoons raw cream
4	tablespoons raw milk
2	ounces fresh mango
1	teaspoon unheated honey

Blenderize all ingredients together in a 12-ounces jar on medium speed for 10 seconds. Pour into popsicle-mold and freeze for 5-8 hours.

ALTERNATIVES 1: Substitute other fruit, such as peach, nectarine, or berries.

ALTERNATIVES 2: Substitute raw coconut cream for raw cream.

Pies

Ambrosia Coconut Cream Pie, Miniature

2 Servings

CRUST
2   ounces raw walnut, or pecan halves
2   teaspoons unsalted raw butter
1/2   teaspoon unheated honey

FILLING, all ingredients room temperature
1   non-steamed date
4   ounces fruits or combination of fruits

TOPPING
2   ounces COCONUT CREAM
1   egg
1   tablespoon unsalted raw butter
1   teaspoons unheated honey, (optional)

Crust: Blenderize walnuts, butter and honey in a 4-ounces jar on medium speed using pulse-action for 5 seconds. Butter bottom and sides of 4-inch glass or ceramic pie-dish. Flatten mixture evenly on to bottom of dish and chill in refrigerator for 15 minutes while making Filling.

Filling: Remove stone from date and chop date. Blenderize chopped date, 2 ounces fruit together in a 4-ounces jar on high speed until creamy. Slice or dice remaining fruit, unless berries, and fold fruit into Filling mixture. Pour and spread evenly over crust and chill in refrigerator for 20 minutes.

Topping: Blenderize chilled coconut cream, butter, honey and egg in an 8-ounces jar on medium speed for 15-20 seconds. Pour coconut cream over chilled Filling and spread evenly. Chill pie in refrigeration for 30 minutes to firm coconut cream. You could save some of the cut fruit from the Filling to make a pattern over the chilled and firmed coconut cream.

Ambrosia Coconut Cream Pie

10 Servings

CRUST
1	**cup walnuts, or pecans halves**
2	**tablespoons unsalted raw butter**
1	**tablespoon unheated honey**

FILLING, all ingredients room temperature
6	**non-steamed dates**
2	**cups fruits or combination of fruits**

TOPPING
8	**ounces COCONUT CREAM**
4	**tablespoons unsalted raw butter**
2	**raw eggs**
1 to 2	**tablespoons unheated honey, (optional)**

Crust: Place walnuts, butter and honey in food processor and blend until ingredients form into a ball. Butter bottom and sides of 8- or 9-inch glass pie-dish. Spread nut mixture. Then flatten evenly on to the bottom of pie-dish and chill in refrigerator for 15 minutes while making Filling.

Filling: Remove stones from dates and chop dates. In a blender, blenderize chopped dates and 1/2 cup fruit (room temperature) together in an 8-ounces jar on high speed for 20-30 seconds, until thick.

Slice or dice remaining fruit, unless berries, and fold into Filling mixture. Pour and spread evenly over crust and chill in refrigerator for 20 minutes.

Topping: Place chilled coconut cream, eggs, butter and honey in food processor and blend for 20-30 seconds. Pour coconut cream over chilled Filling and spread evenly. Chill pie in refrigeration for 30 minutes to firm coconut cream. You can save some of the cut fruit from the Filling to make a pattern over the chilled and firmed coconut cream.

ALTERNATIVE TOPPING: 1 egg only, instead of two, and add 1 1/2 ounces fresh lime or lemon juice, or a combination of lemon and lime juices. Place chilled coconut cream, egg, butter, honey, and lemon and/or lime juices in food processor and blend for 20-30 seconds. Follow the rest of instructions for Topping above.

Ambrosia Cream Pie

10 Servings

CRUST
1	cup raw walnut halves
2	tablespoons unsalted raw butter
1	tablespoon unheated honey

FILLING
6	non-steamed dates
2	cups fruit, or combination of fruits

TOPPING
15	ounces raw cream
1 to 2	tablespoons unheated honey, (optional)

Crust: Place walnuts, butter and honey in food processor and blend until ingredients form into a ball. Butter bottom and sides of an 8- or 9-inch glass pie-dish. Spread nut mixture and flatten evenly on to the bottom of the pie-dish. Chill in freezer for 15 minutes while making Filling.

Filling: Remove stones from dates and chop dates. In a blender, blenderize chopped dates and 3/4 cup fruit in a 12-ounces jar on high speed for 20-30 seconds until thick.

Slice or dice remaining fruit, unless berries, and fold into Filling mixture. Pour and spread evenly over crust and chill in freezer for 10 minutes.

Topping: Blenderize 5 ounces cream and 2 teaspoons honey in an 8-ounces jar on low speed until it is fluffy and stiff. Repeat two more times, each time with 5 ounces cream and 2 teaspoons honey in an 8-ounces jar. Remove pie from freezer and top with whipped cream. You can save some of the cut fruit from the Filling to make a pattern over whipped cream. Let stand in refrigeration for 2 hours.

ALTERNATE TOPPING: Add 2 tablespoon fresh lime or lemon juice, or a combination of lemon and lime juices, to cream and honey. Blenderize as stated above. You can save some of cut fruit from the Filling to make a pattern over whipped cream.

Ambrosia Cream Pie, Miniature

2 Servings

CRUST
2	**ounces raw walnut halves**
2	**teaspoons unsalted raw butter**
1/2	**teaspoon unheated honey**

FILLING
1	**non-steamed date**
4	**ounces fruit, or combination of fruits**

TOPPING
4	**ounces raw cream**
2	**teaspoons unheated honey, (optional)**

Crust: Blenderize walnuts, butter and honey in a 4-ounces jar on medium speed using pulse-action for 5 seconds. Butter bottom and sides of 4-inch glass or ceramic pie-dish. Spread nut mixture and flatten evenly on to the bottom of the pie-dish. Chill in freezer for 10 minutes while making Filling.

Filling: Remove stone from date and chop date. Blenderize chopped date and 2 ounces fruit in a 4-ounces jar on high speed for 10-15 seconds until thick.

Slice or dice remaining fruit, unless berries, and fold into Filling mixture. Pour and spread evenly over crust and chill in freezer for 10 minutes.

Topping: Blenderize cream and honey in a 4-ounces jar on low speed until stiff. Top Filling with whipped cream. You can save some of the cut fruit from the Filling to make a pattern over whipped cream.

Banana Cream Pie

10 Servings

CRUST
1	cup raw walnut halves
2	tablespoons unsalted raw butter
1	tablespoon unheated honey

FILLING
2	eggs
6	non-steamed dates
3	bananas
8	tablespoons unsalted raw butter
2	drops organic vanilla extract, (optional)

TOPPING
15	ounces raw cream
1 to 2	tablespoons unheated honey, (optional)

Crust: Place walnuts, butter and honey in food processor and blend until ingredients form a ball. Butter bottom and sides of an 8- or 9-inch glass pie-dish. Spread nut mixture and flatten evenly into the bottom of pie-dish. Chill in freezer for 15 minutes while making Filling.

Filling: Remove stones from dates and chop dates. In a blender, blenderize eggs, 1 drop vanilla extract, chopped dates, 1/2 banana (break into small pieces) and butter (room temperature) together until thick.

Slice 2 1/2 bananas lengthwise into halves. Slice laterally into 1/8-inch pieces. Fold bananas into Filling mixture. Pour and spread evenly over crust and chill in freezer for 20 minutes.

Topping: Blenderize 5 ounces cream and 2 teaspoons honey in an 8-ounces jar on low speed until it is fluffy and stiff. Repeat two more times, each time with 5 ounces cream and 2 teaspoons honey in an 8-ounces jar. Remove pie from freezer and top with whipped cream. Let stand in refrigeration for 2 hours.

ALTERNATE TOPPING: Add 3 tablespoons fresh lime juice to cream and honey. Blenderize as stated above.

Banana Cream Pie, Miniature

2 Servings

CRUST
2	ounces raw walnut halves
2	teaspoons unsalted raw butter
1/2	teaspoon unheated honey

FILLING
1	egg
1	non-steamed date
3/4	banana
2	tablespoons unsalted raw butter
1	drop organic vanilla extract, (optional)

TOPPING
3	ounces raw cream
2	teaspoons unheated honey, (optional)

Crust: Blenderize walnuts, butter and honey in a 4-ounces jar on high speed using pulse-action for 5 seconds. Butter bottom and sides of 4-inch glass or ceramic pie-dish. Spread nut mixture and flatten evenly on to bottom of pie-dish. Chill in freezer for 10 minutes while making Filling.

Filling: Remove stone from date and chop date. Blenderize chopped date, egg, vanilla extract, half of 3/4 banana (break into small pieces), and butter (room temperature) together in an 8-ounces jar on high speed until thick.

Slice remainder of banana lengthwise into quarters. Slice laterally into 1/4-inch pieces. Fold banana into Filling mixture. Pour and spread evenly over crust and chill in freezer for 10 minutes.

Topping: Blenderize cream and honey in an 8-ounces jar on low speed until fluffy and stiff. Top Filling with whipped cream.

Pumpkin Pie?

(Tastes like it!)

8 Servings

3	ripe persimmons
6	non-steamed dates, remove stone and chop
3	tablespoons unheated honey
1	cup raw walnut halves
2	tablespoons unsalted raw butter
15	ounces raw cream

Crust: Place nuts, 2 tablespoons butter and 1 tablespoon honey in food processor and blend until ingredients form into a ball. Butter 6-inch glass pie-dish. Evenly distribute crust on plate and press firmly. Place in freezer while making Filling.

Filling: Blenderize half of chopped dates and 1 1/2 persimmons in a 12-ounces jar on high speed for 40 seconds. Repeat with remaining dates and persimmons in another 12-ounces jar.

Remove curst from freezer and pour in persimmons mixture. Return to freezer while making Topping.

Topping: Blenderize 5 ounces cream and 2 teaspoons honey in an 8-ounces jar on low speed until it is fluffy and stiff. Repeat two more times, each time with 5 ounces cream and 2 teaspoons honey in an 8-ounces jar. Remove pie from freezer and top with whipped cream. Let stand in refrigeration for at least 8 hours.

Pumpkin Pie, Miniature

1 Serving

3/4	**ripe persimmon**
1	**non-steamed date, remove stone and chop**
3	**teaspoons unheated honey**
2	**ounces raw walnut halves**
2	**teaspoons unsalted raw butter**
3	**ounces raw cream**

Crust: Blenderize nuts, 2 teaspoons butter and 1 teaspoon honey in a 4-ounces jar on high speed using pulse-action for 5 seconds. Butter the bottom and sides of serving bowl. Evenly distribute crust on bottom of bowl and press firmly. Place in freezer while making Filling.

Filling: Blenderize chopped date and persimmon in an 8-ounces jar on high speed for 20-30 seconds until thick. Pour into chilled piecrust. Return to freezer while making Topping.

Topping: Blenderize raw cream and honey in an 8-ounces jar until it is fluffy and stiff. Remove pie from freezer and top with whipped cream. Let stand in refrigeration for at least 6 hours.

**** SALAD ****

Bland-Fruit Salad

1 Serving

1/2	avocado, cut into wedges
6	circular slices raw cucumber
3	circular slices raw zucchini, crookneck or sunburst squash
1	stalk cauliflower tops
1/2	tomato, cut into wedges
2	sliced mushrooms
1	serving of any of the sauces in this book
2	tablespoons red onion, (optional)

Arrange ingredients on a plate or in a bowl and eat with or without a sauce.

** PICKLES, PICKLED PEPPERS & GINGER **

Pickled Ginger

10 Serving

6	ounces thinly sliced fresh ginger
4	tablespoons raw apple cider vinegar
3	tablespoons whey, or natural mineral water
1	tablespoon unheated honey

Blenderize vinegar, whey or water and honey together in an 8-ounces jar on medium speed for 10 seconds. Add ginger slices and cap. If necessary, add more whey or water to cover ginger slices. Marinate for 24 hours in refrigeration. It will keep in refrigeration for about 2 months.

Pickled ginger may be mixed with unsalted raw butter, raw cream, raw coconut cream, olive oil or flax oil and eaten with any meat, red or white.

Pickled Peppers (Pimentos)

10 Servings

1	red bell pepper
1	yellow bell pepper
1/2	cup raw apple cider vinegar
1	cup natural mineral water
1/2	teaspoon unheated honey

Blenderize 1/2 cup water, vinegar and honey in a 16-ounces jar for 5 seconds at medium speed.

Seed and dice peppers, and place in a 16-ounces jar with vinegar/honey/water. If more water is need to cover peppers, add it now, cap and gently turn jar upside down and back several times. Let stand in refrigerator for 24 hours. It will keep in refrigeration for 2 months. If recipe is too much for use in 2 months, divide each ingredient by half and use an 8-ounces jar.

Dill Pickles

10 Servings

4	pickling cucumbers
1/2	cup raw apple cider vinegar
1/2	teaspoon unheated honey
2	tablespoons fresh dill weed
1/2	cup natural mineral water

Blenderize vinegar, honey, dill and 1 ounce water together in an 8-ounces jar for 10 seconds on low speed.

Slice cucumbers lengthwise into quarters. Slice the quarters into halves horizontally. Stuff cucumbers in a 16-ounces jar, pour in blenderized mixture into jar. If more water is needed to cover cucumbers, add it now. Cap and gently turn jar upside down and back several times. Let stand in refrigerator for 24 hours. It will keep in refrigeration for 2 months.

ALTERNATIVE: Add garlic or ginger slices, or any other spice before adding water to cover cucumbers.

Sweet Pickles

10 Servings

4	**pickling cucumbers**
1/2	**cup raw apple cider vinegar**
3	**tablespoons unheated honey**
1/4	**cup natural mineral water**

Blenderize vinegar, 1 ounce water and honey together in an 8-ounces jar for 10 seconds on low speed.

Slice cucumbers lengthwise into quarters. Slice the quarters into halves horizontally. Stuff cucumbers in a 16-ounces jar, pour in blenderized mixture into jar. If more water is needed to cover cucumbers, add it now. Cap and gently turn jar upside down and back several times. Let stand in refrigerator for 24 hours. It will keep in refrigeration for 2 months.

ALTERNATIVE: Add garlic or ginger slices, or any other spice before adding water to cover cucumbers.

Chapter 15

Remedies
and
Natural Topical Beauty Recipes

Primal Facial® Body Care Cream

As well as facial and body skin cream, this is an all-in-one fantastic Sunscreen, Suntan and Sunburn lotion, burn, abrasion and cut salve.

2	ounces raw cream
2	ounces unsalted raw butter
2	ounces raw COCONUT CREAM
1/4	teaspoon unheated honey
1/4	teaspoon royal jelly
1	teaspoon fresh lime juice
1	teaspoon fresh ginger juice

Stir lime juice into coconut cream and let stand for 10 minutes. Then, warm all ingredients in an 8-ounces jar, capped with blender washer/blades/base, immersed in a bowl of mildly hot water for 5 minutes. Blenderize on medium speed for 5 seconds. Rub into skin. Wipe away any excess 20 to 30 minutes after applying on skin. It must be kept refrigerated.

This skin cream feeds the skin and helps prevent and slowly remove lines and wrinkles with regular application. It works for the entire body. In all empirical tests, it acted on ALL participants as both a sunscreen and tanning lotion.

Applying the skin cream liberally to a cut, scrape or abrasion helps to prevent excessive scabbing and the dryness that results from scabbing, and helps heal the wound without scarring. Liberally applied and left on, the skin cream slowly dissolves scabs that have already formed.

During tests for sunscreen potential, some participants thought that they had burned because they were so red. The next mornings there was no burn or soreness, and no one pealed. As a suntan lotion, participants who normally did not tan tanned.

Moisturizing/Lubrication Formula Drink

1 to 2   raw eggs
2 to 4   ounces unsalted raw butter or coconut cream
1 to 2   tablespoons lemon juice
1 to 2   teaspoons unheated honey

All ingredients should be room temperature. Warm all ingredients in an 8- or 12-ounces jar, capped with the blender washer/blades/base, immersed in a bowl of mildly hot water for 5 minutes. Blenderize on medium speed for 10 seconds. It is most effective when consumed with, or shortly after, a meat meal.

Most bodies are so starved for healthy raw fat that when they get fat, the organs, blood, glands and nervous system consume it. The lymph, bones, joints, connective tissue and skin continue to starve and shrivel with dryness unless we get enough fat. We cannot eat enough fat to supply all that our bodies' need after years of cooked food. However, this formula helps rush fats into the body so that lymph, bones, joints, connective tissue and skin receive some wonderful fats. Because fats are utilized for so many functions, I suggest eating this recipe almost daily.

To make this recipe sound appealing to both sexes, I gave it two names. When I give this formula to women, I call it the Moisturizing Formula. When I give it to men, I call it the Lubrication Formula.

Pain Formula

3 to 4   level tablespoons refrigerated fresh soft bee pollen
1 to 2   ounces no-salt-added raw cheese
1   MOISTURIZING/LUBRICATION FORMULA DRINK

Add pollen to the Moisturizing/Lubrication Formula above prior to blenderizing, and then blenderize. Eat cheese as you drink the formula. Usually, this formula reduces pain 80-100% within 10 minutes to several hours. It is 5-10% less effective if the cheese is not eaten.

Natural Deodorant

Splash and rub fresh lemon juice under armpits and wipe. It is effective in most cases of very strong body odor. A drop of ginger juice rubbed into underarms usually creates an alluring fragrance. One tablespoon of ginger and/or mint juices per quart of green vegetable juices also helps body odor.

Natural Antiperspirant

Cut pieces of lemon rind and pulp (no juice) and dry it in the sun for 30 days. Grind into a powder. Brush it into armpits that have been splashed and rubbed with lemon juice and wiped.

Diet During Symptoms Of Cold, Flu Or Severe Pain

1/2 to 1 pound fowl
2 to 3   MOISTURIZING/LUBRICATIONS FORMULA DRINK
         (preferable), see page 146
   or 2 to 3 MILKSHAKEs, see page 57
1   SMOOTHIE, see pages 58-59
This daily diet should be followed until symptoms have subsided and normal functions resume.

Lemon Throat Lozenge

4   ounces butter
2   tablespoons fresh lemon juice
3   tablespoons honey
2   teaspoons fresh ginger root juice or 2 tablespoons grated
         fresh ginger root

Warm all ingredients in an 8-ounces jar, capped with blender washer/blades/base, immersed in bowl of mildly hot water for 5 minutes. Blenderize on medium speed for 5 seconds. Enjoy 1-2 teaspoons, retaining the mixture in the mouth for as long as possible, swallowing a tiny amount at a time. That will coat the throat over a 1- to 4-minutes period, allowing it to absorb into and coat the throat.

Toothpaste

Mix ¼ teaspoon sun-dried clay, 2 tablespoons raw butter or raw cream and 2 drops ginger or mint leaf juices. Good for 5 tooth-brushings. Keep refrigerated.

Constipation, Chronic, Relief

Chronic constipation indicates that intestinal bacterial levels are much too low. Sixty to eighty percent of our bowel movements should be bacteria not fiber on a raw diet. E. coli is the main bacterium in our colons responsible for proper bowel movements. Eating high raw meat supplies the body with natural bacteria destroyed by cooking and internal polution. Those bacteria help reduce waste and decay in the body. Eating moist clay and/or HIGH MEAT (see blow) helps build intestinal bacteria responsible for healthy bowel movements. These suggestions may be the only long-term solutions: 1 teaspoon of moist clay eaten every other day, and 1 marble-sized portion of high meat eaten once a day for 14 days, then once a week for as many months as it takes to resolve constipation. Also, read Constipation Remedy, Temporary, and read pages 174-177 in this book. Other constipation remedies are in my book *The Primal Diet; We Want To Live, Volume 2*, see Constipation.

Depression, Chronic, Relief

can be consistently alleviated by eating HIGH MEAT (see below). It often causes an attitude shift in people with "entitlement" issues, that is, the segment of society who feels the world owes them. Worries usually settle. Normally, those effects last from 2 to 60 days. People who suffer severe depression eat high raw meat as often as every day. One client feels so happy, he eats 1 cup each day. People who have cancer help reverse it by eating high raw meat. If suffering intestinal, neurological or lymphatic cancer, high raw chicken is more favorable.   See pages 170-174.

High Meat Recipe
(red meat, seafood, and fowl)

Place 1 volume-pint of raw meat, chopped into bite-sized pieces, into a glass quart (32 ounces) jar; equal air- and meat-space. Place *Ball* jar lid on jar tightly and place in the refrigerator. I suggest three jars be prepared; one with raw red meat, one with natural raw fowl and one with ocean wild-caught raw fish. Every 3 to 4 days take the jars outdoors, completely remove lids and wave the jars in the air to exchange the air inside each jar. Return lids to jars, tighten and return to refrigeration. After 4 weeks, you may begin to eat one marble-sized piece once or twice every week. There are approximately 17 stages of bacterial developments. Airing the meat is required to progress bacteria through the stages. If you don't replace the air in the jar every 3 to 4 days, the bacteria stages will not progress. If you go on a trip, when you return, recommence airing the meat so that it will resume progress through all of the bacterial stages.

To make eating high raw meat easier, take it outside (or your home will stink for up to 36 hours), close the nostrils with fingers or swimmer's nose clip, and eat. You can swallow it without chewing but chewing makes it more effective to lift spirits. The odor is terrible, but the texture is palatable. If you do not like the after-taste, rinse mouth with lemon or lime but do not swallow the lemon or lime. Lemon and lime are antibacterial, especially lime. If you swallow the citrus juice, it is likely that you will experience little benefit. I have eaten high raw meat that was aged up to 1-year old with excellent benefits when I needed it.

If suffering depression or chronic constipation, I suggest eating high raw meat twice a week. Do NOT eat large amounts of high meat while on a weight-loss cycle.

Constipation Remedies, Temporary

Temporary relief may be obtained by soaking 2 ounces raw Chia seeds in 5 ounces of good water for 24 hours. The water turns to a gelatinous consistency. Stir seeds and gel into one entire Moisturizing/Lubrication Formula Drink and eat like cereal once a day as necessary.

Besides those above and in my book *The Primal Diet; We Want To Live, Volume 2*, here is an more aggressive remedy. Because the combination prevents proper digestion, the body moves this remedy through the intestines quicker. This is not suggested for regular use but for emergencies only. Usually, this remedy drunk once is enough. Only 10% of the test-subjects had to drink two or three within 24 hours.

3	**ounces stone-pressed olive oil**
2	**ounces raw milk**
2	**ounces raw unpasteurized apple cider vinegar**
2	**ounces unheated honey**
2	**ounces fresh lemon juice**

It is best to drink all of it as quickly as possible. Occasionally, stomach cramps result. I suggest placing a hot-water bottle on the stomach and breathe deeply and slowly. Never use an electric heating pad. Electrical devices produce electromagnetic fields that unfavorably alter cellular structure. Never use microwave packs; they irritate cellular membranes.

Volume Three

The Science Of Living Healthfully

Chapter 16
Our Digestive Abilities

We want the raw foods that have proved to digest efficiently and healthfully. We want those that transform into substances that balance, build, grow, regenerate, reproduce cells, lubricate, soothe, cleanse and fuel us. We cannot utilize that which we cannot digest properly and in healthful balance.

Our intestines are 2½ times shorter than most herbivores[8]. We have only one stomach, while herbivores have 2-4 stomachs. Herbivores have nearly 60,000 times more enzymes than we have to disassemble cellulose (plant fiber) to obtain the fat and proteins from vegetation and grain. Vegetable fiber passes through an herbivore's digestive system in about 48 hours. In our digestive tracts, vegetables complete their journey in 24 hours. Only a fraction of the cellulose is digested. Sixty-five percent of the protein and fat are undigested.

On a primarily cooked diet, eating whole, raw vegetables usually prevents constipation. They supply enzymes and fiber needed to counter some of the putrefaction and the resultant tendency toward constipation that occur with cooked food in our digestive tracts. Contrarily, on a raw diet, eating whole raw vegetables more than once every 2 weeks often causes over-alkalinity of our digestive tracts. Alkalinity destroys or neutralizes the acidic bacteria that digest all meat, dairy and eggs, frequently causes loss of appetite for raw meat, and causes constipation. We do not digest raw whole vegetables well. Normally, they are not part of a health-giving diet for humans.

---

[8] Animals who consume mainly vegetation, such as cows, horses, deer and sheep.

Our gastrointestinal tract is not like that of birds. Birds can eat a lot of grain (seeds) and digest it with their gizzards. We do not have a gizzard or an alternative way of eating grain that is health-giving. We cannot properly digest grain for cellular reproduction and healing, even if sprouted. Sprouted grains are vegetables. As stated above, we do not digest vegetables well. Germinated seeds contain enzyme suppressors that prevent proper protein digestion, utilization and assimilation, causing protein deficiency.

Our intestinal shape is like some frugivores (primates) who mainly eat fruit. However, when humans eat a lot of fruit they incur health problems, such as osteoporosis, tooth degeneration, anxiety, dryness, diabetes, hyperactivity, attention-deficit disorder (ADD), attention-deficit hyperactivity disorder (ADHD), over-emotionality and temperature sensitivity. Unlike pure frugivores and herbivores, we mainly have an acidic digestive tract, including acidic bacteria that facilitate the prevention and reversal of cancer. More than a little raw high-carbohydrate fruit over-alkalinizes the intestines. Intestinal over-alkalinity destroys proper protein and fat digestion and suppresses appetite for raw meat, and can make raw meat repulsive to us. That destroys our ability to combine many foods and impairs the natural acidic environment of our bowels. A sugar-rich environment caused by high-carbohydrate fruits results in fungal problems, such as candida and other yeast infections. Eating more than a little fruit causes severe fat and protein deficiencies. In women, that often causes bloating and menstrual cramps.

Carnivores, such as cats and dogs, mainly eat meat. Our digestive juices are most similar to carnivores. In their stomachs, the hydrochloric acid concentration is 15 times greater than in humans so that they digest meat in 10 hours, which accommodates their very short intestines. Humans, however, produce an equal amount of hydrochloric acid throughout the stomach and intestines combined, allowing raw meat and other raw animal products to digest easily and efficiently in our much longer digestive tract within 16 hours. (Cooked meat takes 24-36 hours to digest accompanied with putrefaction, heterocyclic amines, acrylamides and lipid peroxides not found in the digestive tract when raw meats are eaten.) Our teeth are designed for cutting and crushing meat with the help of our dexterous hands.

Lastly, there is the omnivore, such as the pig, who eats everything. Our digestive tract is similar in size and action to a pig's, but 35 years of experimentation with food has taught me that limiting the human diet to mainly a raw carnivore diet results in healthier and happier well-being.

Chapter 17
What Does Cooking Do To Nutrients In Food?

A major problem with food-science is that its scientists view nutrients in food in only two categories, good and destroyed. That is like viewing people as follows: A person who is vibrant, strong and athletic is considered good, useful and functional; a person who is weak and tired is considered good, useful and functional; a person who is crippled is considered good, useful and functional; a person who is comatose is considered good, useful and functional; and a person who is dead is considered destroyed.

Nutrients that are mutilated are not very useful or functional for creating and maintaining health. Yes, the weak, crippled and comatose people are alive but how productive can they be toward accomplishing the daily chores? How many weak, crippled and comatose people have you asked to dig ditches and lumberjack?

I have observed that no matter how slight the damage to nutrients, that digestion, utilization and assimilation are impaired. Science fails to acknowledge that truth. I have found that health is poorly affected when people eat food that artificially reaches a hot-temperature as low as 93° F (34° C), and cold-temperature as high as 40° F (4° C).

Research throughout the world shows that heat-treatment of food alters, damages, or destroys many vitamins at standard pasteurization temperatures from 140° to 161° F (59° to 71° C). All enzymes are destroyed at prolonged artificial temperatures from 122° F (49° C). Consider, as I stated above, that the artificial temperature that weakens or cripples some nutrients, including vitamins and enzymes is as low as 93° F (34° C). The loss of mineral utilization due to cauterization[9] is significant.

Cooking protein-foods, including all meat, above 104° F (39° C) produces toxins. Higher cooking temperatures create more dangerous toxins, such as heterocyclic amines (caustic compounds) that have proved to be carcinogenic in laboratory animals.[10] Cooked protein is difficult to utilize for cellular reproduction, regeneration and healing.

---

[9] Cauterization is when heat or a caustic substance burns a substance to the point where it is relatively impervious and unable to exchange molecules to sustain or promote activity.

[10] "Analysis of cooked muscle meats for heterocyclic aromatic amine carcinogens", Knize MG, Salmon CP, Mehta SS, Felton JS; Mutat Res, 1997, May 12; 376(1-2):129-34.

"Cooked casein promotes colon cancer in rats, may be because of mucosal abrasion", Corpet DE, Chatelin-Pirot V; Cancer Lett, 1997, Mar 19; 114(1-2):89-90.

"Mutagenic activity of heterocyclic amines in cooked foods" Felton JS, Knize MG, Dolbeare FA, Wu R; Environ Health Perspect, 1994, Oct; 102 Suppl 6:201-4.

"Cancer risk of heterocyclic amines in cooked foods: analysis and implications for research", Layton DW, Bogen KT, Knize MG, Hatch FT, Johnson VM, Felton JS; Carcinogenesis, 1995, Jan; 16(1):39-52

"Exposure to heterocyclic amines", Wakabayashi K, Ushiyama H, Takahashi M, Nukaya H, Kim SB, Hirose M, Ochiai M, Sugimura T, Nagao M; Environ Health Perspect, 1993, Mar; 99:129-34.

"Occurrence of mutagens in canned foods", Krone CA, Iwaoka WT; Mutat Res, 1984, Nov-Dec; 141(3-4):131-4.

"The formation and occurrence of amino acid pyrolysates and related mutagens in cooked foods", Massey RC, Dennis MJ; Food Addit Contam, 1987, Jan-Mar; 4(1):27-36.

"Food-derived mutagens and carcinogens", Wakabayashi K, Nagao M, Esumi H, Sugimura T; Cancer Res, 1992, Apr 1;52(7 Suppl):2092s-2098s.

Heating fat above 96° F (36° C) causes toxic alterations, including lipid peroxides (oily oxidizing compounds) that have proved to be carcinogenic. Cooked fats cannot exchange ions or molecules properly. An example: If the body forms, from cooked fats, an improper or incomplete lubricant to protect the arteries, the fat hardens and arteries become brittle after many years, especially from heated vegetable oils.

Stockholm University in cooperation with Sweden's National Food Administration (a government food safety agency) showed that cooking carbohydrate-rich foods, such as bread, cake, biscuits, crisps, donuts and French fries, produces high quantities of acrylamides. The British Food Standards Agency confirmed the Swedish findings that acrylamides cause gene mutations leading to a range of cancers in rats, including breast, uterine, adrenal and scrotum cancers. The British study revealed levels of acrylamides 1,280 times higher than international safety limits in fried supermarket potatoes, chips and crisps, such as Walkers crisps, Ryvita crackers, Kellogg's Rice Crispies and Pringles crisps. Acrylamides increase damage to the nervous system and affect fertility.[11] The Swedish report showed that the average potato chip contains up to 25 times more acrylamides than the top level allowed in drinking water by the World Health Organization (WHO). Heating food destroys many health-giving properties and produces disease-causing toxins that accelerate bodily deterioration associated with aging processes.

A deleterious array of effects from eating cooked and processed foods commonly occur within the body. Molecules degrade and repeatedly collide, causing divalent-bonding that results in the formation of "new chemical composites". Mucoid-plaque layers often form in intestines, lymph and blood structures. A tremendous increase in white blood cells floods the digestive tract (leukocytosis) trying to harness and neutralize

---

"An experimental approach to identifying the genotoxic risk by cooked meat mutagens", Loprieno N, Boncristiani G, Loprieno G; Adv Exp Med Biol, 1991; 289:115-31.

[11] "World alert over cancer chemical in cooked food", Robert Uhlig, Food Correspondent, News.telegraph.co.uk, (18 May 2002), United Kingdom.

toxins. Up to 50% of cooked protein eaten coagulates and becomes unutilizable and cross-linked. Body-food synergism is corrupted. High levels of methionine result, promoting the creation of homocysteine that initiates atherogenic free-radicals.[12] Extremely caustic waste products result, causing cumulative congestion that clogs the body's circulatory systems. Putrefactive and mutagenic bacteria proliferate, producing more caustic waste and byproducts (intestinal toxemia) that disrupt normal actions of the intestinal flora, and are absorbed into blood, lymph and nerves, causing systemic toxemia. Lipofuscin accumulates in the skin and nerves, including brain. Water in food is reduced from 100% utilizable to an average 20% absorbable and 8% utilizable. Often, excessive overeating or anorexia results because nutrient-deficient food is unsatisfactory for our bodies' requirements. Bio-electromagnetic energies within food are lost rather than conveyed cellularly.

The following analogy applies to many nutrients, including fats and minerals that are destroyed by cooking and other food-treatments: Clay is malleable, pliable, and able to foster growth of bacteria and plants. When fired, clay becomes hardened and life-deprived. When cooked, nutrients in food become hardened and life-deprived. Bones, for example, become brittle, like glass, and impervious to salivary secretions when they are cooked. If cooked bones splinter and lodge in a pet's throat, the splinters may lacerate and embed, causing the animal to choke to death. Its saliva cannot penetrate the cauterized bone. If raw bones splinter, the animal's saliva dissolves it within minutes and the animal does not suffer any significant suffering or damage.

Most often, animals develop disease from being fed cooked and processed food, especially food-manufacturing byproducts and waste, hormones, antibiotics, vaccines and chemicals. If we become ill from eating diseased meat, such as cattle infected with mad cow disease, the blame should not be directed toward bacteria but toward the cattlemen who grow and produce diseased animals for us to eat. The USDA and FDA is also responsible; they fail to protect us, making regulations that hurt

---

[12] Accumulations of homocysteine have been linked to heart problems.

the people and make profits for agribusiness. Animals fed cooked and processed byproducts and wastes, chemicals and drugs, become diseased if they live long enough. They are usually slaughtered before disease is apparent. The products from those animals should only be eaten if a healthier/better quality of meat is unavailable.

Chapter 18
Other Forms of Nutrient Destruction

Cooking and processing are not the only ways to damage food. All methods to eliminate bacteria and parasites and preserve food (pasteurization, irradiation, freezing, ascorbic acid and other chemical additives and washes) destroy nutrients and create toxins. They rob us of nutrients and pollute us.

Research proved that exposing food to high intensity gamma radiation affected the activity of key enzymes and caused the depletion of radiation-sensitive, essential nutrients, including the amino acids l-cysteine, l-histidine, and l-tryptophan, vitamins C, E and K, B1, B 2, B3, B6 and B12, folic acid, an omega-3, 6 and 9 unsaturated essential fatty acids. Some irradiated minerals in food become toxically radioactive. Radiation-mutated nutrients advance aging. Irradiation destroys the health-giving properties of food and poses public and environmental hazards.

Isolated ascorbic acid, whether used as a preservative or "Vitamin C" supplement, robs the blood of fat, causing nerve lesions throughout the body, including the brain and spinal cord. That often causes irritability and depression. Hydrogen peroxide burns cells, destroys bacteria and neutralizes many viruses. All chemicals have proved side-effects, immediate or long-term. Chemical destruction of helpful virus and bacteria in our food results in poisoning, often causing anger and/or depression. Freezing food alters, damages, or destroys most enzymes and damages many vitamins. In animal tests, animals fed exclusively uncooked frozen meat developed severe skin problems, including mange. The other group fed the same diet of the same meat but unfrozen remained healthy and vibrant. Therefore, food that is heat-treated, freeze-treated, dehydrated, chemically preserved, irradiated or processed in any manner that destroys nutrients and creates toxins is not raw or health-giving.

Chapter 19
Is The High-Cholesterol Problem A Myth?

On this diet, sometimes cholesterol levels radically increase. That is normal and healthful. As the body removes stored toxic cholesterol, it often moves it through the blood and out the urine. The combination of new health-giving cholesterol and the old toxic stored-in-the-body cholesterol accounts for the increase. The presence of both cholesterols in high amounts has not posed harm or threat in any case that I have observed for the last 32 years. When enough raw fats are eaten, the toxic cholesterol leaves our bodies through our urine, bowels and skin without re-absorption into the body. When on this diet, a radically high cholesterol level in the blood is a wonderful indication that toxic cholesterol has been removed from tissues and is being eliminated.

Most often, a high intake of <u>raw</u> fat lowers cholesterol levels in six weeks, but in a few cases, high cholesterol levels continue for years while health increases. Therefore, I suggest that we completely ignore cholesterol levels when eating raw fat. Raw fats continue to exchange ions as long as they are in a warm living body. Raw animal fats do not cause hardening of the arteries, osteoporosis, or brittle bones. Cooked and processed fats cause those diseases, especially processed vegetable, nut and seed oils.[13]

---

[13] *The Cholesterol Myths; Exposing the Fallacy That Saturated Fat and Cholesterol Cause Heart Disease* by Uffe Ravnskov, MD, PhD; ISBN 0-9670897-0-0; (2000)

Chapter 20
Should I Take Supplements To Replace Missing Nutrients?

Processed food is full of food-byproduct toxins, mutilated minerals, proteins, fats and carbohydrates, and destroyed enzymes and vitamins. Research has proved that those foods, when enriched with vitamins, enzymes and other expensive supplements produce the same diseases that processed and cooked foods produce.[14, 15] Manufacturers sell us the false notion that enrichment of their processed foods resolves deficiencies created by processing and makes their product the greatest food on Earth.

All vitamin supplements are merely portions of the vitamin, like bran is to a grain. They are not what we are led to believe they are and will not do what we believe they will do.[16] Supplements are always drugs and not food, even if they are derived from food. Extraction-processes alter nutrients and poison them. Once a nutrient is isolated from its bioactive form and extracted, it is no longer bioactive. If it is not in food form, it is not raw or bioactive. Pill, powder and liquid supplements are only 2-12% utilizable, and are 88-98% waste that will be isolated and eliminated, leeching and usurping our bodies' innate vital nutrients.

The worst-case example of a toxic supplement is Vitamin E. Most Vitamin E is the byproduct of the film-development and film-process industry. Because the chemical waste (tocopheral) is similar in molecular structure to natural Vitamin E (d-alpha tocopheral), it is called Vitamin E and sold as a supplement. In reality, those manufacturers make profits instead of paying fortunes for the hazardous disposal of their toxic waste. In other words, profiteers make money by seducing us into purchasing and ingesting toxic waste. Vice versa, foods rendered into waste

[14] *The Milk Book* by William Campbell Douglass, Jr., M.D. (1997).
[15] *The Real Truth About Vitamins & Antioxidants* by Judith A. DeCava, MS, LNC; A Printery, Massachusetts, 2001.
[16] Ibid.

products after vitamins and other nutrients are chemically extracted, are then made into foods, such as chips and cereals, or animal fodder. That subject alone is worth a shelf of books. Even natural Vitamin E has to be either heat-processed or solvent-extracted. Heat-processing destroys Vitamin E and solvent-extraction causes destruction and low-grade poisoning.

Consider doctors' advice to take iron supplements if iron level in the blood is below what they think it should be. The iron-level concept is a seatbelt of the medical/pharmaceutical industry to hold people into the supplement-vehicle from which they profit. I have seen repeatedly that iron levels are individual and have nothing to do with particular diseases or vitality. Diseases always have their roots in multiple deficiencies and gross toxicity. See Baby Food/Infant Formula, page 43, for a case history of an infant who was diagnosed by a medical doctor with anemia and retardation and who was prescribed iron, mineral and vitamin supplements.

Mineral absorption and utilization depends upon ion and electrolyte activity and exchange. When food is cooked or processed, ions and electrolytes are neutralized and often separated from minerals and nutrients. Many of the minerals become free-radicals, including iron, causing cellular destruction and degeneration, often resulting in infections. Iron supplements are never ionically or electrolytically active. They are ineffective and harmful. Free-radical iron that is absorbed into tissue but not utilized cellularly often rusts in the body causing severe degeneration. The only way to assure that iron is properly absorbed and utilized, is to eat raw foods that contain bioactive iron. A bioactive iron-rich food is raw meat that strengthens blood, liver, adrenals, pancreas, gallbladder, spleen and muscles.

Massive free-radicals and other toxins store extracellularly and/or intercellularly. They cannot be converted to cellular food. Affected areas of the body malfunction or rupture and become sites of disease.

In the case of very debilitating and painful intestinal Crohn's disease, several major toxins accumulate in the intestines: Free-radicals, acrylamides, AGEs, and heterocyclic amines and other toxic protein-byproducts and wastes accompanied by cellular low-fat levels, and caustic bilious byproducts. Those toxins destroy the intestines' natural bacterial environment. That corrupts digestion. Specific vitamin-deficiencies include Vitamins K and U. Supplemental consumption of those vitamins is rarely effective because of processing. However, the ingestion of raw green cabbage juice has proved to be effective toward healing 90% of ulcerative cases.

Why Do Supplements Seem To Work?

Most pill, powder and liquid supplements create a toxic high similar to the high created by caffeine, causing a rise of hormones, such as adrenaline, that buffer, hide or arrest symptoms without resolving disease and without effecting cure. Decades of research proved that the body manufactures adrenaline in response to injury and most poisons that enter the blood stream. Hormonal rushes and cessation of symptoms are usually interpreted and marketed as increased health. Therefore, people think falsely that supplements work to increase health and cure disease. Like medications, supplements are drugs.

Left to the body's natural abilities with the present level of toxicity, most people on cooked diets will heal cancer and other disease 60% of the time. Many of those cures follow colds, flu, meningitis or pneumonia (natural detoxifications). Any test for any product or diet that shows less than 60% recovery is not only ineffective but also harmful.

Our vitamin, enzyme and mineral supplementation should be fresh raw green vegetable juices.

We will redefine and restructure healthcare.

Volume Four

Health Or Disease?

Chapter 21
Origins of Modern Medicine

In the 1870's, Louis Pasteur proved that heat-processing slowed food spoilage and lengthened the shelf life of mold-damaged wine. He saved vineyard owners from financial loss and ruin, but he condemned wine drinkers to seasons of toxic wine produced from unhealthy crops of grapes.

Pasteur presumed that fungus and bacteria caused disease. He failed to realize that an unhealthy crop succumbed to fungus and molds. Rather than looking to enrich the soil to generate healthy grapes, he attacked the fungus and mold that were symptoms of the unhealthy crop. Diseases, he surmised, originate from constant types of microbes attacking the body from outside.

Contrary to Pasteur, his contemporary, Dr. Antoine Bechamp, 1816–1908, claimed that disease originates from within the body because of the destruction of cellular integrity by toxic food and pollution. He contended that all microbes were beneficial, some for cleansing, some for maintenance and others for regeneration, but that none were responsible for causing disease.

I suppose that because we are a warring society, we ignored Bechamp and embraced Pasteur. Maybe it was easier for us to believe that we could recognize and battle invading forces rather than consider changing our life styles. Regardless, modern medicine's justification for microbial wars is based on speculation, fear and pseudoscience.

Louis Pasteur made the "germ theory" famous but he killed it on his deathbed. Many reports said that some of his dying words were:

Pathogens are not the problem. The environment in which and on which pathogens feed is the problem of disease.

That means that the cause of disease is the quality of our air, food and all substances with which we come in contact.

Louis Pasteur's dying words were lost because philanthropists, people in government and pharmaceutical houses lobbied and funded the research to plan and fight a war against germs (microbes). Those who joined the microbial war were intellectuals, mainly academics, who were excited by the opportunity to prove the germ theory and once and for all to win a battle against disease. However, instead of conducting experiments to prove or disprove any validity to the theory, they accepted the theory to be as true as the law of gravity.

Through Pasteur's work, the new medical scientists of the time gained respect and quickly seized the opportunity to root in academia. Consequently, our science does not understand how disease develops. Medical science is obsessed with studying cellular particles without understanding the basic nature and relationship of the body holistically. They established an arsenal of weapons. They created drugs and tools of diagnoses, surgery and radiation. The original intention to defeat disease became rhetoric. The new intention became profit.

Medical science readily wages war in our bodies, treating the symptoms of disease with drugs, surgery, chemotherapy, radiation and machines. This treatment of symptoms, rather than the causes of disease, has proved to imbalance body chemistry and has filled our bodies with toxins. Most often, those toxins cause loss of quality of life and more disease. The foundation and structure of modern medicine is disease, not wellness. Humanity suffers from disease because we do not focus on rational cure and prevention.

We have libraries based on Pasteur's point of view, so let's look at information that supports and proves the accuracy of Dr. Bechamp's work. In the early 1900's, German zoologist Günther Enderlein observed through a powerful dark-field microscope, hundreds of tiny moving beings in blood that entered into union with organized bacteria. Enderlein stated that in the serum of all people and warm-blooded animals, there are living microorganisms that often are called the "bug factory". He properly named them endobionts, meaning "internal life". Enderlein saw what Bechamp believed existed: That all microbes beneficially partake in a natural developmental cycle, changing into bacterial and fungal phases, including those misnamed as "pathogens". It is a modern-day tragedy that Bechamp's work has not been funded and tested rigorously.

Chapter 22
Modern Medicine

Most medical doctors have studied 0 to 16 hours of nutrition in premedical and medical school. Whether we consider Sloan Kettering, Johns Hopkins, Mayo, Beth Israel, or the Cleveland Clinic, the knowledge base of food and nutrition, its efficacy, and the funding of testing are virtually non-existent. If modern medicine does not understand the cause of disease, how can it elevate our health? We cannot be medically treated without compromising our health and most often the quality of our lives.

To illustrate how irrational much of modern medicine is, consider that today's biotechnology has produced 791 anticancer agents. None of them are designed to eliminate the causes of cancer. Trillions of dollars have been spent on cancer, yet medicine has not invented any effective "therapy" that does not have serious side-effects. Modern medical therapies fail miserably, with an overall survival rate of approximately 17% beyond 5 years.

Through the media, the pharmaceutical industry and scientific community keep us believing that someday they will sell us a magic potion that will create a super immune system and a disease-free environment in the human body. Although that scenario is extremely improbable, people continue to fund and believe in them. More likely, we will reflect from a future time upon the human body's poisoning by today's medical therapies similar to the way we viewed the practice of bloodletting in the 20th Century. Future science will probably condemn today's paradigm of modern medicine for being exactly what it is: Ignorance, lack of education, and unwillingness to fund natural research into the cause and prevention of disease. The change is likely to be difficult because cancer is big business, trillions of dollars each year.[17]

Today's medical science tries to prevent microbes rather than pollution from entering our bodies. It attempts to cleanse Nature's ubiquitous microbes from the body and environment rather than cleanse us of toxins. They annihilate rather than nurture our cells with the liveliest nutrient- and bacteria-rich raw food. Our mechanical sciences are brilliant but our life-sciences are stuck in a quagmire of delusion, pride and greed. Nurturing is the wisest approach to prevent and reverse disease. Nurturing maintains and/or restores the highest quality of a fully enjoyable rich life, even if we live in simplicity.

Chapter 23
Discovering How To Live Disease-Free

Let's look at some animals who lived their entire lives without degenerative disease. Dr. Francis Pottenger, M.D., demonstrated in his tests with 900 domesticated cats, over a decade, that cats developed strong bones when they were fed raw dairy and raw meat, without the consumption of bones.

---

[17] "AN EPIDEMIC of Deception; We Can't Trust The Cancer Establishment; An Interview With Dr. Samuel Epstein" by Derrick Jensen; *The Sun magazine;* March, 2000.

Also, he found that sick domesticated cats with osteoporosis reversed the disease when they were fed raw meat and raw milk. Edward Howell repeated the same clinical tests with rats and received the same results. The records we have of <u>animals that have lived without degenerative disease shows that they enjoyed a non-toxic environment and ate a raw diet that suited their digestive abilities.</u>

In the 1860's, dental decay first appeared among the Eskimo people, occurring only in Eskimos who lived in white man's colonies, eating breads and sugar. The first case of cancer among Eskimos occurred in 1934. Like dental decay, cancer appeared only among second- and later generations of Eskimos who ate breads, sugar and cooked food for nearly a century.

In his book *Cancer:Disease Of Civilization?*, Chapter 14, "The Longevity Of 'Primitive' Eskimos," Vilhjalmur Stefansson stated that there was only one community of Eskimo reported to have had a short life span. That report has been used to propagandize that Eskimos lived short lives because of their predominately raw animal-food diet. In all other reports, "primitive" Eskimos lived as long as we do, with the same percentage of people exceeding the age of 100 years. Eskimos who ate their normal raw diet enjoyed teeth so strong that they chewed on bones during evening congregations. Osteoporosis only occurred in Eskimos who ate cooked, refined foods. If you placed average civilized humans of the 21st Century in the Alaskan environment, equipped with the same skills and required to live as the primitive Eskimo did, most would die within one winter's climatic exposure.

Chapter 24
Dawning Of Disease

Two factors cause the rampant, modern progression of afflictions such as cancer, diabetes, osteoporosis, obesity and heart disease. The first factor is eating cooked and/or processed food that is devoid of unadulterated nutrients and full of the toxic byproducts of cooking, pesticides and other chemicals.

The second factor is environmental pollution. The industrial and chemical revolutions have created over 6,000 bizarre foreign chemicals that our bodies have not succeeded in processing as food or air. Toxic accumulations within our bodies cause more deterioration. Some chemicals cause immediate death, but most cause the gradual degeneration that leads to poor-quality health and disease. The dithiocarbamates are a group of fungicides including mancozeb, metiram, zineb and ziram which have a metabolite called ethylene thiourea (ETU). This breakdown product is a known endocrine-disruptor, carcinogen, mutagen and teratogen, and can become concentrated when food is processed and heated. In other words, if you cook a vegetable that has been sprayed with mancozeb (the most common), you will be increasing the amount of that dangerous metabolite.[18]

In New Zealand, over 60% of the 138 samples of fruits and vegetables analyzed for dithiocarbamates in the latest total diet

---

[18] *Age and Susceptibility to Toxic Substances,* Calabrese, E.J. 1986, New York: John Wiley & Sons.
"Anthropological approach to the evaluation of preschool children exposed to pesticides in Mexico", Guillette, E.A.et al 1998, *Environmental Health Perspectives* 106: 237-347. In: Watts, M. 2000: Endocrine disruption: a case for the precautionary approach. *Soil & Health* March/April.
Eating Safely in a Toxic World: What really is in the food we eat, Kedgley, S. et al 1998, Penguin NZ.
"Effect of a mixture of 15 commonly used pesticides on DNA levels of 8-hydroxy-2-deoxyguanosine and xenobiotic metabolizing enzymes in rat liver", Lodovic, M. et al, 1994, *Journal of Environmental Pathology, Toxicology and Oncology* 13: 3, pp163-168.
Food Additives. Penguin Books, Millstone, Erik, 1986
Introduction. In: Mourin, J (ed), Nair, K.P. & Mourin, J, 1999, *Warning: Pesticides are Dangerous to Your Health!* Pesticide Action Network Asia and the Pacific, Penang.
Pesticides in the diets of infants and children, Nair, K.P. & Mourin, J, 1999, Washington: National Academy Press.
"The physiological susceptibility of children to pesticides", Whyatt, R., 1993, *Journal of Pesticide Reform* 9:3, pp5-9.

survey contained dithiocarbamates. The 17 fruits and vegetables that ranked highest, in order according to occurrence and mean dithiocarbamate-concentration were broccoli, cabbage, tomato, celery, lettuce, onion, cucumber, apple, orange, mushroom, potato, courgette, kumara, nectarine, pear, capsicum and kiwifruit. Levels are worse in the USA because more chemicals are used.

Chemical risk assessments are generally based on animal tests. Scientists disagree about the reliability of the tests in assessing the effects pesticides will have on humans for a lifetime. Because of the inexact nature of toxicology, precise and unequivocal risk assessments for some substances are difficult. Over time, our knowledge about particular substances increases and technology and testing methods become more sophisticated. The result is that acceptable daily intakes (ADI) become unacceptable, as in the case of the pesticide DDT. As the current concentration of agribusiness-favorable public servants ruling the FDA, USDA and CDC[19] increases, we are more endangered every day.

International regulatory agencies concede that the concept of an ADI is a crude way of assessing toxicity. There is no scientific justification for choosing a safety factor of 100 rather than 75 or even 10. Professor Erik Millstone argued that it is a random guess chosen for political rather than scientific reasons and is nonsense in the real world.[20] We should not be subjected to any level of health-disruptive chemicals.

---

[19] Federal Drug Administration, US Department of Agriculture and Center for Disease Control.
[20] "Pesticides In Food: Why Go Organic, Analysis of New Zealand's latest Total Diet Survey", Alison White, Pesticide Action Network NZ/ Safe Food Campaign, Wellington, NZ, (Millstone 1986).

Chapter 25
Are Bacteria, Viruses and Parasites
Dangerous to Humans?
And Is Microbe Genocide A Rational Pursuit?

Today there are several astute scientists challenging the postulate that bacteria are the threat. Before the Los Angeles County Medical Milk Commission, Dr. Marc Harmon, a dentist, stated that his medical education trained him to blame disease and decay on bacteria and virus. He stated that the genocide of microbes has not reduced dental decay any more than it has reduced disease in general. Disease continues to increase at an astounding rate. Science, medicine and technology have waged a horrific war against microbes, while tooth decay and other diseases continue to overwhelm and devastate our lives. Dr. Harmon concluded that the war against microbes is futile in eradicating disease.

William Campbell Douglass, Jr., M.D., presented numerous scientific reports showing that raw milk is not a bacterial risk, even when abundant with "pathogenic" activity, and that raw milk helps the body develop strong bones free of osteoporosis. (See pages 180-186).

At the University of Utah, John R. Roth, Professor of Biology, studied salmonella for 40 years. He stated that salmonella is mostly reported as a pathogen but lives beneficially as part of the gut flora.[21] He believes that the idea of eliminating it is absurd because salmonella is distributed widely. Rarely does it get across the gut wall. When it does, it is simply an irritation at the gut wall. Symptoms can range from loose stools to flu-like symptoms. The idea of eradicating microbes like salmonella is ludicrous because they are everywhere, in your nose, mouth, on your skin and pets.

The University of Arkansas for Medical Sciences and the Arkansas Children's Hospital did a study of 50 Arkansas homes

---

[21] *The Great Egg Panic*, LA Times, Jan. 4, 2000.

where salmonella-infected children lived. They found that salmonella was widespread with concentrations in 38% of the homes on unsuspected places, such as doorsteps, vacuum cleaners, refrigerators, and a pet lizard.[22]

The questions we beg to have answered are these: Are the microbes activated in a nontoxic environment? Are the microbes active because they are doing a beneficial job? If they are, they are supposed to be in our bodies. If we change our life style to improve our internal environment, will the microbes still become active?

Los Angeles Times researcher Emily Green wrote that her foray through Salmonella literature from present to the early 1940s revealed that what was perfectly legitimate *speculation* in the last 12 years by CDC doctors concerning the possible origin of Salmonella enteritis transmogrified into fact once their speculations were stated in political reports. CDC speculation concerning Salmonella enteritis remains unproved.[23] Ms Green stated that most of what appears in scientific and medical journals is guesswork. That explains the recent reversal over cholesterol in eggs - that egg-cholesterol is now benign, or may be favorable. They do not know. Yet, the CDC is the most influential health department in the world. Its doctors influence most of the decisions that affect everyone. As I stated, they are driven by fear, speculation and junk science.

Chapter 26
Should Microbes That Are Considered Disease-Causing But, Actually, Are Disease Eliminators, Be A Part Of Our Optimal Diet And Lives?

During the last 25 years, I have seen hundreds of "incurable", life-threatening, degenerative diseases reverse and heal by

[22] "Salmonella Bacteria Often Lurks Close By"; *Richmond Times Dispatch*, July 19, 1999.
[23] *The Great Egg Panic*, LA Times, Jan. 4, 2000.

people eating a raw diet that was mainly raw animal foods. I have experienced a continuing series of events in which degenerative tissue (cancer, etc.) disappeared within days, weeks or months following bacterial, viral and parasitic infestations. My body's environment has become increasingly healthier over time because of the invaluable assistance of microbial activity, including pathogenic. And yet, science and the medical industry consider me greatly "at risk".

In a test project, Jon Monroe, Director, New Science, tried "to avoid diseases caused by viruses. The assumption was that viruses were pathogens and should be avoided." But, after employing techniques to prevent virus production in test individuals, each of the subjects became and remained clinically depressed for one year. When viruses were allowed to flourish again, symptoms of depression disappeared, and colds and flu returned. Monroe realized that it was better to have detoxifications in the form of periodic colds and flu rather than constant depression. They play a crucial role in health, symbiotically.[24, 25]

The microscience that studies "pathogens" is relatively new (50 years) and flawed. Newer research (20 years) has been and is being performed, proving that "pathogens" are responsible for the reversal of cancer, and possibly for cancer prevention. As part of her doctoral studies at the University of Toronto, Canada, Dr. Sara Arab injected verotoxin, a bacterial byproduct from E. coli, directly into human malignant brain tumors. After a single injection, the verotoxin completely dissolved both the tumors and their blood vessels within 2-7 days.[26] Dr. K. Brooks Lowe of

---

[24] Symbiosis: Unlike organisms living harmoniously and beneficially together.

[25] Strange Attractor, Volume 2, Number 1, A News Letter of Alternative Science and Medicine; http://www.newscience.santa-fe.nm.us/strange.htm

[26] "Verotoxin Induces Apoptosis and the Complete, Rapid, Long-Term Elimination of Human Astrocytoma Xenografts in Nude Mice" by S. Arab, J. Rutka, and C. Lingwood; *Oncology Research*, Vol. 11, pp. 33-39, 1999.

Yale University reported that researchers used salmonella to reverse cancer.

Many universities in Canada have been developing cancer treatment using viruses to penetrate cancer cells and dissolve them for decades. Many tests have been successful. Oncologist Don Morris at Calgary's Tom Baker Cancer Centre said, "It's common to hear that cancer patients who pick up a virus get a regression of their disease." Several of the universities that have jumped on the viral bandwagon are Havensack Medical School in New Jersey, Stanford is using the common cold virus, Harvard is using a herpes virus, Duke University is using a weakened polio virus, Mayo Clinic is using a measles virus. The projected retail price of an injection to the patient will be $8,000. I suggest that we get colds or flu, eat high meat regularly and pay nothing.

Even though virus therapy has been successful, many of the patients now suffer with chronic viral symptoms. That is what happens if you treat the disease without understanding and correcting the cause. Dr. Patrick Lee from Duke University observed that viruses penetrate and dissolve unhealthy cells. So, the question to be answered is: What makes cells unhealthy? For the answer, read pages 166-168.

Robert and Michele Root-Bernstein cited in their book *Honey, Mud, Maggots and Other Medical Marvels*, that for hundreds of centuries, various worldwide cultures ingested bacteria and molds for medicinal purposes. The Hunza (one of the world's longest-lived people), certain Eskimo, Fulani, Masai and Samburu tribes of Africa regularly ingest "pathogens". The Hunza and Fulani drink salmonella and E. coli daily in their raw milk. Eskimo tribes bury their meat in hides for up to six weeks. The bacteria-infested meat, called "high meat", is ingested to elevate the mood, eliminate aches and pains, and increase endurance. None of the primitive tribes have degenerative diseases. A number of raw food eaters in the USA and worldwide regularly ingest bacteria-infested food for those purposes. The Chinese successfully used "century" eggs for remedies and disease prevention, and as an aphrodisiac. Century eggs are decomposed eggs aged up to 25 years with high-bacteria concentrations and molds.

The supposition that the elderly, infants and ill people are more susceptible to harm from "pathogens" is speculation and false. I have observed that in most cases in which so-called "at-risk" individuals ate bacterially rich, aged and decaying raw food, they regained health of their bowels, digestion, glands, sanity, and in many cases, reversed disease. It worked favorably in all situations with only 6 people in 32 experiencing minor loose bowels, nausea and/or vomit. Those people considered their temporary discomfort well worth the long-lasting beneficial results. Content tests of diarrhea and vomit showed high levels of a variety of toxic substances that were not part of the food or byproducts. The tests results indicated that those toxins already existed in the patients' bodies and were being flushed from their bodies.

Parasites are the most feared of "pathogens". Parasites, too, have a symbiotic relationship with our bodies. They consume and digest tremendous quantities of degenerative tissue in short periods. Joel Weinstock, a gastroenterologist who heads a research team at the University of Iowa stated that we are the first population to be without gut worms. He asked six patients with very painful, intractable inflammatory bowel disease to drink the eggs of Trichurissuis, a whipworm parasite normally found in the intestines of pigs. Within two weeks, five of the six patients entered remission for up to five months. The patients begged for more parasites. Weinstock noted that intestinal problems are increasing in animals because they are kept too clean. Pigs and monkeys raised in sterile pens and cages are getting diseased.

Parasites afford us the quickest process of organic detoxification. Parasites are a problem only if an individual does not readily reproduce cells. Meaning, they do not replace the degenerative cells consumed by parasites. In such a case, ulcers could result and fester, causing numerous problems including death. Eating raw meats with raw fats prevents ulceration by providing the nutrients necessary to support quick cellular

reproduction following the tremendously beneficial detoxification precipitated by parasites.

If an individual eats foods or chemicals that cause gross
destruction and decay (degenerative tissue), she or he will be
less able to tolerate parasitic and bacterial detoxifications. If he
or she eliminates chemicals, pollution, and destructive foods, he
or she will stop adding to the problems that make parasitical and
microbial detoxification necessary. To facilitate the removal of
degenerative tissue, people can eat "high" meat, meaning that
the meat is high in bacteria, and that it makes people's spirits
high. For high-meat recipe, see page 149.

Although the germ-theory has been predominantly disproved,
modern medicine continues to uphold it.

Chapter 27
Then Why Are There So Many Reports About
Bacterial Food-Poisoning?

There have been medical reports that stated microbial food-
poisoning as cause of death. In most cases, the reports described
symptoms of anaphylaxis,[27] or drug-damage/poisoning, rather
than bacterial food-poisoning. On a rare occasion, someone has
died from dehydration and/or excessive bleeding caused by a
ruptured stomach or bowel from violent vomit or diarrhea.
"Pathogens" are sometimes found in the presence of diarrhea
and vomit but have not been proved the cause.

Any foreign substance that causes traumatic allergic reactions
causes anaphylaxis. Anaphylaxis is a very common response to
injected antibiotics and vaccines. The people who were reported
as having died of bacterial food-poisoning probably died of the
medical treatment from antibiotics and/or other medication. E.

---

[27] Anaphylaxis is a severe allergic reaction to anything, usually
medication.

coli 157:H7 has been blamed for Hemolytic Uremic Syndrome (HUS) and kidney failure, but the claim has not been proved. The treatment of bacterial infection involves the use of drugs containing poisons, such as thimerosal (mercury). Research has proved that mercury causes HUS-like symptoms, kidney and neurological damage. The antibiotic Cipro has been linked to kidney degeneration. Drugs damage kidney cells setting the stage for virus and bacteria to dissolve or consume them. The medical treatments for bloody diarrhea are probably the major cause of HUS and kidney failure. Of the hundreds of "at risk" people on the Primal Diet who experienced vomit and bloody diarrhea, not one suffered glandular or organ damage. They did not take any medication or medical therapy. Also, antibiotics affect heart, lungs and central nervous system. Most often, it is the drug treatment that causes some deaths in cases diagnosed as bacterial food-poisoning. Scientific inquiry needs to be thorough. However, that research is not likely to occur because it would open a flood of lawsuits against doctors, hospitals and pharmaceuticals.

People are afraid to eat pathogens, bacteria and parasites even though all wild animals eat them without ill-consequence. Even if "pathogens" were a real danger, they are here among us. A few people may be harshly affected by "pathogens" but most will not. As some people will die during common colds and automobile accidents, most will not. The attack on, kangaroo-trial and lynching of "pathogens" in our foods, bodies and households are scientifically wrong and dangerous.

Immunity is likely to arise if we ingest bacteria the way all other animals do. But people are afraid to eat bacteria called pathogens, especially E. coli. No other animal except the civilized human washes itself or its food before eating. All animals eat feces full of E. coli except civilized man. No animal experiences bacterial food-poisoning except us. Do wild animals naturally eat small amounts of feces for the bacteria and parasites as a cancer preventative? The tests at all of the universities mentioned, indicate that they do. Edward Howel's experiments proved that rats who ate cooked and processed food and naturally ate their feces had less severe diseases and lived a third longer than those who did not eat their feces.

A friend of mine, who I will call Jean, suffered from chronic fatigue syndrome for 8 years, cancer of the right breast, hipbone, left kidney and adrenal gland (before we met to discuss the diet). She was lucky to work 6 hours per week. She progressed on the Primal Diet slowly for 2½ years. Jean's body completely softened and dissolved all of her many breast tumors but the others showed little shrinkage.

Finally, because her cancer was so advanced, I shared with Jean the results of tests using E. coli and other bacterium to dissolve tumors. Jean asked where she could get the bacterium. I explained that E. coli is natural to bowels and could be consumed in feces from any healthy animal. I explained that other bacteria could be grown on high meat. She did not want to wait to grow bacteria on high meat, so she pursued feces.

Jean consumed 2 ounces by volume the first time from a healthy herbivore. That is not much, considering that some tribal members eat an entire load from a water buffalo at one sitting. However, within two months, all of her tumors shrunk by 15%. Since that time, she has consumed some feces from gopher, goats, sheep, chicken and duck. She is cautious with the quantity she eats and has not consumed more than half a cup at a time. She did not incur much diarrhea. Jean's tumors have shrunk 60% in the 2 years since she began eating a little feces every 3 to 4 months. Most tumor-shrinkage occurs in the 4 weeks following ingestion of feces or high meat.

Jean is completely physically and mentally active. She is vigorous. Now, she lives rather primitively on a self-sustainable farm. She performs hard and continuous labor daily. She loves having her health and new-found strength.

We must measure which is the greater risk: Is it more perilous to eat raw food, get healthier and accept rare minor diarrhea and/or vomit, or to eat cooked and processed food, develop deficiencies, collect toxicity, develop disease, and experience occasional-to-frequent, mild-to-severe, diarrhea and vomit?

When I develop detoxifications in the form of vomit or diarrhea, my chances of living are greater if I eat properly, stay completely away from terrorist medical advice and treatments, and let it run its course, as with a cold or flu. Usually, any intestinal bleeding easily stops within hours of drinking 8 ounces of fresh, raw, green cabbage juice.

Chapter 28
Why the Hysteria Over Bacteria, Viruses and Parasites?

The assumption and false premise is that microbes labeled "pathogens" are always harmful and must be eradicated. Health-department officials are in the cerebral dark ages. They are prejudiced against microorganisms labeled "pathogen", and have based their raw food restrictions on prejudicial correlations, erroneous statistics and pseudoscience. Most doctors, scientists and health department employees maintain one-sided views of the "pathogen" and "bacterial food-poisoning" controversies. They ignore existing data that proves pasteurization does not provide food safety nor prevent disease, but <u>causes</u> disease. Their adherence to the mind-set against the virtues of microbes called pathogens does not make rational sense and produces poor judgment in policy-making.

Peoples' fears of loss, injury and the unknown have always been at the heart of medicine and food regulation. Consequently, we attack our bodies and food as if they were inherently dangerous. Our collective approach in this life, then, has been to make war within and outside of ourselves to survive and thrive. It has proved to be a futile approach to health and life.

The virtues of attaining zero exposure to "pathogens" cannot be proved to exist, yet people believe in pursuing that goal. Zero exposure to "pathogens" is not possible anyway, because they are everywhere. Making threshold-extrapolations to generate quantitative-risk estimates is pseudoscience. Using the impossible criteria of zero exposure to bacteria in order to estimate risk is pseudoscience. Existing regulatory policy is based on a better-safe-than-sorry premise. In the real world of everyday practicalities where common-sense decisions are needed, better-safe-than-sorry is simply ignorance and a morally bankrupt posture.

There is nothing "better" about the illusion of "food safety" when it results in people using scapegoats - "pathogens" - in place of scientifically verifiable causes of actual harm. The conviction that one individual's right to absolute protection should preempt the well-being of others is poor social planning, especially if the protection of the minority harms the majority.

Government regulators are not responding to what is actually harming people. They pander to imaginary issues that frighten people and themselves. We must be brave against the FDA, USDA, CDC and health-department officials and employees. We do not need to fear political or social pressure, third party judgments, or the disinterest of our peers when discussing this paradigm. This is vital information to our individual and collective lives. It is devastating that we have virtually lost our raw food supply that is our primal link to optimal health. Government regulators must be educated and laws criminalizing and/or penalizing the sale of raw food must be reversed immediately.

To change the laws in your city, county and state, see the Right To Choose Healthy Food[28] website: www.rawmilk.org

Chapter 29
Follow The Money

The last equation in this problem is the vested money and corporate interests concerned with product shelf life, medics, pharmaceuticals and agri-chemicals that fuel microbe-hysteria.

---

[28] *Right To Choose Healthy Food* is a not-for-profit organization based in Santa Monica, California. See page 186-189.

The food industry wants pasteurization, chemical washes, antibacterials and irradiation because their products will have a longer shelf life, reducing their costs by slowing spoilage. They care much more about their products, costs and profits than they do about our health. Almost all of them encourage government officials to pass laws mandating compulsive pasteurization and irradiation, yet industry tells us that the government is to blame for industry producing and supplying more toxic products.

***

> *"Pathogens" are to the body what vultures, crows and ants are to the Earth. They are a few of the Earth's janitors. They find carcasses and eat them. Without the Earth's janitors, our air would be in jeopardy of becoming toxic gas in which animals could not thrive. "Pathogens" are our bodies' helpful, organic, inner-ecological recycling organisms that help us thrive.*

Chapter 30
Bacterial Summary:
Does a Recipe for Optimal Health Include "Pathogens"?

As our houses must be taken apart to be renovated after becoming dilapidated, so must our bodies. According to Dr. Elnora Van Winkle, retired biochemical neuroscientist from the Department of Psychiatry at New York University's School of Medicine, "pathogens" are the clean-up and demolition crews for degenerative conditions.[29] They appear as a response, not as the cause. "Pathogens" respond to decay within the body, reversing or preventing disease that is more serious. They are the first stage of the cure, the cleansing stage. Eliminating pathogens, such as salmonella, campylobacter and E. coli, and parasites forces decaying tissue to remain in the body, endangering the inner body environment. Our bodies gradually get sicker.

We must comprehend that bacteria are absolutely everywhere. Our bodies rely upon microbes for every healthy

---

[29] Letter To The Editor, *Health Science Magazine*, February 1999.

function. As in all wars, there are untold casualties. Lands are blown to pieces, people are maimed, poisoned, devastated and exterminated. Financial resources of the majority of people vanish in explosions and are vaporized by technology. Recovery for people and the environment is long and hard, taking decades, if it occurs at all. The maimed live maimed. The dead are dead.

When we make war on germs, the battlegrounds are our bodies. We are the casualties, our cells, ourselves. Our finances are drained and exhausted on a war we cannot win. Such wars enrich the wallets of doctors, chemists, investors, employees of pharmaceutical houses, retail outlets, hospitals, insurance companies, health departments and every industry that provides supplies and services all of them.

Imagine spending 1/6 of our resources and 1/3 of every day attacking a necessary torrential storm that cannot be stopped without long-term devastation. Imagine losing everything we own to support that unnecessary and futile war. That is what we do when we try to live pathogen-free by attacking our bodies rather than changing our life-styles. If we do not want disease and their symptoms, we simply need to live a life-style that does not make our bodies into huge feeding lots for microbes.

We have the answer to what makes us sick and that is the biological degeneration that results from eating cooked and processed foods, and exposure to industrial, environmental and therapeutic pollution, including medications. The more waste and pollution we have in our bodies, the more symptoms of degeneration we suffer. Should we teach how to prevent and reverse disease, or should we spend our lives in fear, fighting futile microbial wars? My choice is to live without disease.

Chapter 31

Infant Safety, Health Benefits, Propagandized False Risks From Feeding Raw Milk, And The Harm Of Feeding Infants Pasteurized And Other Processed Milk.

Consistent with most doctors' modern beliefs, they prescribe food and therapies for infants and children that have created disease in our children. Unscientific propaganda issues from them constantly. They say that raw milk is dangerous for infants, causing bacterial food-poisoning and death without one credible scientific experiment to support that theory. I present to you many published reports from the first 5 decades after pasteurized and processed milks were introduced to the public. They prove that feeding infants pasteurized or processed milk is dangerous and causes disease. They prove that feeding infants raw milk is safe and healthful.

In 1984, William Campbell Douglass, Jr., M.D., presented considerable clinical evidence to the world that drinking pasteurized milk resulted in degrees of osteoporosis and bone malformation, diabetes, and many other diseases. Also, he provided clinical evidence from the same sources that drinking raw milk reversed osteoporosis, bone malformation, diabetes and many other diseases. He cited the findings of studies documented at the following universities and clinics: Harvard, Princeton, Cambridge, Dartmouth, Tufts, the Washington University School of Medicine, the University of Georgia Dairy Science Department, the Ohio State University School of Agricultural Chemistry, and Mayo Clinic of Minnesota.

He presented testimony confirming those findings from the following medical journals and publications: *The Lancet, JAMA, World Cancer Research Fund* journal, *American Journal of Clinical Nutrition, New England Journal of Medicine, British Medical Journal, Consumer Reports, Consumer's Union,* Hartford's prestigious *St. Vincent's Hospital Report, Certified Milk Magazine, American Association of Medical Milk Commission Report, Milk Industry Foundation Report,* and *The Price Pottenger Nutrition Foundation Newsletter.*

Colic is a concern with infants who are fed pasteurized milk. One of every five babies suffers colic. Pediatricians learned in the early 1900s that pasteurized cows' milk was often the reason. A more recent study linked pasteurized cow's milk consumption to chronic constipation in children. Those researchers observed that pasteurized milk consumption resulted in perianal sores and severe pain during defecation, leading to constipation.[30]

Dr. Francis Pottenger, Jr., MD observed several infants. They were born of mothers known to be hypothyroid. Prior to the birth of those infants, the mothers had given birth to children within three years. Each of the previous children suffered asthma, infantile rickets, and skeletal underdevelopment. In one experiment, the baby girl that had been fed formulas since birth was always sickly. The formulas included powdered milk, pasteurized milk, boiled milk, boiled certified milk and canned milk. She suffered severe gastric distress during her infancy. When she was 8-months young, she developed asthma. She was undersized, considering her parents had large builds. Contrarily, the healthy child was breast fed from birth. The mother drank raw milk and lived under excellent health-promoting conditions.[31]

Dr. Weston Price, D.D.S., proved fifty years ago that processed milk leads to disease and premature death.[32] He also showed that processed food, such as pasteurized milk, causes poor development of facial bones. Nizel of Tufts University reported that decayed teeth were four times more common in pasteurized-milk-fed babies as opposed to raw-milk-fed babies.

Dr. A. F. Hess wrote in his abstracts that pasteurized milk was an incomplete food. He proved that many infants developed scurvy on a diet of pasteurized milk. The form of scurvy took some months to develop and was termed subacute. He considered it not only the most common form of scurvy but also the one that passes most often unrecognized.[33] The infants were cured of scurvy when raw milk was substituted. Regarding his

[30] Iacono G, Cavataio F, Montalto G, et al. "Intolerance of cow's milk and chronic constipation in children" N Engl J Med 1998;339:110-4.
[31] "Clinical and experimental evidence of growth factors in raw milk", Certified Milk, January, 1937.
[32] Nutrition and Human Degeneration, Price-Pottenger Nutrition Foundation, La Mesa, California.
[33] Infantile Scurvy. III. Its influence on growth (length and weight), Am. J. Dis. Child., August, 1916.

tests, he stated that, taken in conjunction with the fact that they fed the same number of infants on raw milk as pasteurized milk, cases of scurvy did not develop in infants on raw milk. He stated that their test-results were sufficient to warrant the deduction that pasteurized milk is a causative factor in infant scurvy.

Dr. Pottenger proved there is deficiency disease similar to Vitamin C deficiency (scurvy) that can be cured by giving an endocrine product that contains no Vitamin C. He proved that raw milk naturally contains that endocrine nutrient and that pasteurized milk does not. He proved that raw milk reversed and prevented scurvy.

Stefansson, an anthropologist working for the U.S. government, reported that an artic sea-captain who ingested high amounts of Vitamin C did not reverse his scurvy. After the captain ate raw meat for several days, he completely healed.[34] It was reported in 1942 that grazing cows produced as much Vitamin C as does the entire citrus crop, and that most of it is lost as the result of pasteurization.[35]

In Berlin prior to 1901, rarely was there a case of infant scurvy. In 1901, a large dairy established a pasteurization plant in which all milk was raised to a temperature of about 140° F (60° C). After an interval of months, infantile scurvy was reported from various sources throughout the city.[36] Neumann recorded that he and two other doctors had seen only 32 cases of scurvy from 1896 to 1900. He reported that the number of cases suddenly rose to 83 cases in 1901 and 1902. An investigation was made as to the cause. Pasteurization was discontinued. The number of cases decreased as quickly as they had increased.[37] Neumann also reported that the cases of infantile scurvy were marked by susceptibility to infection, abdominal cramps, nasal

---

[34] Harper's Magazine, November/December, 1925 & January 1936, from the Stefansson Collection, Dartmouth College.
[35] Proc. Nat. Nut. Conf. for Defense, May 14, Federal Sea Agency, pp. 176; U.S. Government Pat. Off., 1942.
[36] Newmann, H., Deutsch. Klin., 7:341, 1904
[37] Ibid.

184 Volume Four   the Recipe for Living Without Disease

diphtheria, furunculosis of the skin, and pneumonia in advanced cases.[38]

Dr. Hess reported that milk-pasteurization that was intended to prevent humans from getting diseases that cows sometimes develop was a waste. He further reported from his observations and tests that infants fed pasteurized milk easily developed common diseases. He stated that deaths from those common diseases should have been attributed to the defective nature of pasteurized milk.[39] Humans do not get bovine undulant fever nor does it naturally transmute into human undulant fever. There is no credible data that proves otherwise.

Dr. J.E. Crewe, from the Mayo Foundation, Minnesota, reported the therapeutic uses of raw milk in 1923. He stressed, from his experiments, that the key-factor was the feeding of *raw* milk. He stated that while raw milk is widely used and recommended as an article of diet, physicians seldom use it as an agent in the treatment of disease. For 15 years, he employed the raw-milk-diet treatment in various diseases and obtained "uniformly excellent" healing results. Dr. Crewe witnessed rapid improvement in his patients with advanced cases of pulmonary tuberculosis when he utilized raw-milk therapy. That was ironic, considering that tuberculosis of the time was blamed on raw milk. Hippocrates used raw milk to cure tuberculosis.

Research by Johns Hopkins University and the University of Maryland found that raw milk contained 2½ times more IgG enzyme than pasteurized milk. In the presence of higher levels of IgG, rotavirus that cause diarrhea in infants is not produced.

In 1923, at St. Vincent's hospital in Philadelphia, concern arose for the high death rate among infants from gastroenteritis. Dr. Paul B. Cassidy, M.D., recommended raw milk instead of pasteurized milk. The raw critics panicked, predicting a catastrophic increase in infant deaths. The death rate in infants

---

[38] Ibid.
[39] Hess, A. F., "Recent advances in knowledge of scurvy and the antiscorbutic vitamin," J.A.M.A., April 23, 1932.

from gastroenteritis quickly fell by 94%, from a high of 89 in 1922 to less than 5 per year.[40]

Destin was a child who developed asthma as an infant on baby formulas, suffered near-fatal attacks yearly, grew frail, weak, underdeveloped, extremely small for his age, and was on regular medication. Dr. Douglass treated him, at the age of nine, by feeding him raw milk. In six weeks, Destin stopped wheezing for the first time in his life. Destin grew rapidly on the raw-milk treatment, living a normal life thereafter.[41]

A Dutch chemist, Willem J. Van Wagtendork at Oregon State College, proved that pasteurized dairy creates calcification and stiffness. He found that guinea pigs with calcification of the tissues could be relieved with raw cream but not so with pasteurized cream. The active health-giving factor is transmuted and rendered ineffective by pasteurization. John Fowler, M.D., Worcester, Massachusetts reported that raw-milk therapy relieved muscle cramps in pregnancy.

There has never been an epidemic proved caused by raw milk. All epidemics from milk were proved to be caused by pasteurized milk. The following list reveals that pasteurized milk products are dangerous. As Dr. Lee explained, pathogens enter unhealthy cells. Pasteurization kills milk cells. Pathogens multiply rapidly in those cells. If someone eats a product that is full of pathogens, the bacteria will proliferate in a body full of unhealthy cells.

Some Outbreaks Attributed to Bacterial Food-poisoning from PASTEURIZED MILK products
- **1945—1,492 cases for the year in the U.S.A.**
- **1945—1 outbreak, 300 cases in Phoenix, Arizona.**
- **1945—Several outbreaks, 468 cases of gastroenteritis, 9 deaths, in Great Bend, Kansas.**

---

[40] Annual Convention, Certified Milk Producers Association, Hotel Roosevelt, New York City, February 8, 1938.
[41] The Milk Book; How Science Is Destroying Nature's Nearly Perfect Food, Wm. Campbell Douglass, Jr., MD, 1996, Second Opinion Publishing, Georgia; pp. 204.

- 1978—1 outbreak, 68 cases in Arizona.
- 1982—over 17,000 cases of *yersinia enterocolitica* in Memphis, Tenn.
- 1982—172 cases, with over 100 hospitalized from a three-Southern-state area.
- 1983—1 outbreak, 49cases of listeriosis in Massachusetts.
- 1984—August, 1 outbreak S. typhimurium, approximately 200 cases, at one plant in Melrose
            Park, IL.
- 1984—November, 1 outbreak S. typhimurium, at same plant in Melrose Park, IL.
- 1985—March, 1 outbreak, 16,284 confirmed cases, at same plant in Melrose Park, IL.
- 1985—197,000 cases of antimicrobial-resistant Salmonella infections from one dairy in California.[4243]
- 1985—1,500+ cases, Salmonella culture confirmed, in Northern Illinois.
- 1993—2 outbreaks statewide, 28 cases Salmonella infection.
- 1994—3 outbreaks, 105 cases, E. Coli & Listeria in California.
- 1995—1 outbreak, 3 cases in California.
- 1996—2 outbreaks Campylobactor and Salmonella, 48 cases in California.
- 1997—2 outbreaks, 28 cases Salmonella in California.

Chapter 32
Losing Our Choices To Live Disease-Free;
A Plea For Help

Health departments are pushing for eradication of pathogens in our food supply. They accomplish that by laws controlling food suppliers. The USDA and FDA, with the help of CDC and congress, has banned us from being able to purchase bottled raw

---

[42] Ryan CA, Nickels MK, Hargrett-Bean NT, et al. "Massive outbreak of antimicrobial-resistant salmonellosis traced to pasteurized milk", JAMA 1987;258:3269-74.
[43] "CDC. Outbreaks of Salmonella enteritidis gastroenteritis -- California", 1993. MMWR 1993; 42:793-7.

fruit and vegetable juices at our local healthfood stores and supermarkets because, they claim, that one girl died from drinking orange juice containing E. coli. The evidence was entirely circumstantial. Nevertheless, they used that incident to scare congress and people into depriving us and our children of another healthy vitamin- and enzyme-rich food source. Coca Cola was pushing for the mandatory pasteurization laws because they own a major juice company. As I said earlier, they want to restrict our resources because they will have little competition if competitors cannot offer a better and cheaper product. Also, because they will experience less product-loss from the mandated processing that lengthens shelf-life.

State health departments have pushed legislation to prevent restaurants and other ready-made-food retailers to cook foods to certain temperatures or else be in violation of the law. With the present trend, soon we will not be allowed to buy any food that has not been completely adulterated. We are being regulated by legislation as to what we are allowed to eat and how it has to be prepared. Most of us rely upon commercial markets for our food. Markets have to follow whatever the health departments demand or they will be shut down and out of business.

We, as the consumers, have few choices. The more restrictive the laws on food and food preparation, the less choices we have. I have watched the laws move in that direction every month for the last 10 years. I have tried as much as possible to stop the momentum but I cannot do much without your help.

Consider that the deck is already stacked against us. Most of the pharmaceutical giants own the major chemical and agrochemical businesses that produce the poisons that are poisoning our bodies and lands.

Consider that, my more recent tests indicated that people eating cooked, non-organic foods are losing their microbe levels. There are so many medications, antibacterials and chemicals, including gaseous, in the environment and food that microbes cannot survive the poisoning. They are becoming as extinct as the firefly. Sooner than we might think, people will be paying for injections of viruses, bacteria and parasites.

Will people be told that they have to have injections of viruses, bacteria and parasites to survive? Who will have kept the FDA- and USDA-certified microbes alive in laboratories? Would it be the pharmaceutical industry that is also the major owners of antibacterial chemicals and agrochemicals industries? If you live in a city, how much will you have to pay because you will not be allowed to get them naturally in your food or environment? Laws went into effect in the year 2002 that restricts transport of soil, seeds and plants. The law states that if the plant you want to transport and grow is not on the list, it will be confiscated and destroyed. If it is on the list and not an approved source, it will be confiscated and destroyed.

Unless we can change those laws together, we may not be able to enjoy a healthy life-style without living on a farm with approved crops and bacteria that only you will be able to eat and not sell. Only cooperative communities, which can establish themselves according to their own laws, will enjoy a natural healthy life-style.

I am the Executive Director for the not-for-profit organization Right To Choose Healthy Food. We battle the government whenever they threaten to deprive us of healthy food with regulations, such as the laws that have been enacted requiring all milk and juices to be pasteurized if they cross any state line. At present, we are battling to reverse those two issues. It takes researchers, lawyers and many resources. Please send generous donations made payable to:

Right To Choose Healthy Food
P.O. Box 176,
Santa Monica, CA 90406-0176.

We need your help and support regularly.

Issues arise quickly in government with little or no notice to the public. Email is the quickest way to contact you and rally your support for unconstitutional laws that deprive us of health and liberty in the name of pseudo-safety. Please help us help you and our children. Send me your addresses, especially an email address. Thank you.

Healthfully,
Aajonus

For information on individualized consults and programs with Aajonus, e-mail or leave a message, speaking slowly, with a fax number. Aajonus wishes that he had more time to answer all of your letters but he is inundated with work. At present, he is fighting for our rights to have raw food and writing 4 more nutritional books: one on detoxification, two of questions and answers from lectures, one on changing food laws, and an update and revision of *The Primal Diet; We Want To Live* (the basic changes are in this book).

Optimal Ways of Living
P.O. Box 176
Santa Monica, CA 90406-0176

e-mail: optimal@earthlink.net
Message: 310-226-7055

A new book giving helpful information about food, nutrition and the Primal Diet will be published every six months for the next 2 years starting January 2006. An audio version of The Primal Diet; We Want To Live will be available in Summer 2006. Also, CD/DVDs will be published by Fall 2006 that shows how to make recipes and use kitchen equipment, and another in which Aajonus presents a workshop on how to live disease-free with more clarity, strength and energy. Notice for all publications will be posted on the website www.PrimalDiet.com.

Index

A

acceptable daily intake (ADI), 168
acid/alkaline balance
    in blood & digestive tract, 30
    in food-combining, 36–37
    fruits and, 30
    raw vegetables and, 151
acrylamides, 117, 153, 155, 161
adhesions (scars), 34
adrenal glands, raw (recipe), 104
Advanced Glycation End-products (AGEs), 32, 117, 161
African Lamb (recipe), 88
aging process, 21, 37, 155
agricultural chemicals, 29-30
alkaline/acid balance. *See* acid/alkaline balance
Ambrosia Coconut Cream Pie (recipe), 134–135
Ambrosia Cream Pie (recipe), 136–137
amino acids, destruction of, 157
anaphylaxis, 174
animals
    E. coli consumption by, 175
    effect of processed foods on, 157
    and Pottenger's raw diet, 165–166
antibiotics, 16, 156, 174-175
Antiperspirant, Natural (formula), 147
Arab, Dr. Sara, 170–171
arterial/intestinal plaque removal (recipe), 55
Asian Spicy Meat Sauce (recipe), 62
asthma, 182, 185
autoimmune inoculation, 18
avocados, combining as fruit, 36

B

baby food recipes, 43, 51–53
    Infant Glandular Booster, 52
    Infant Immune Booster, 52
    Infant Milkshake, 53
    Infant Nervous System Booster, 53
bacteria
    as detoxifying agents, 23
    as disease eliminators, 170–174
    fallacy of war on, 168–169
    false concern over, 18–20, 177–178
    food poisoning from, 174–177, 181, 185
    futility of eliminating, 179-180

C

D

fats, raw
 cholesterol levels and, 158
 daily intake of, 39
 dissolving and binding with toxins, 21, 28
 eaten with fruits, 32–33
 function and benefits of, 28
 optimum temperatures for, 26
 with raw meats to reverse aging, 21–22
 severe bodily shortage of, 146
 toxins produced by heating, 155
feces as healing agent, 176
fibromyalgia, 29
fish, raw, 29
fish/seafood recipes, 105–113
 Ceviche, 107
 Escolar Fresca, 107
 Hot Buttered Salmon, 107
 Oyster Sauce & Pasta, 108
 Oysters Over Cheese, 109
 Salmon with Lemon & Parsley, 110
 Shrimp Passion, 110
 Spiced Salmon, 111
 Spiced Sashimi, 111
 Swordfish Sashimi, 112
 Tahitian Fish, 112
 Thai Ceviche, 113
flax oil, 34
Flu, Cold, Severe Pain (formula), 147
food-combining, 36–37
food-poisoning, bacterial, 174–177, 181, 185
food preparation equipment (listed), 45-46
fowl (white meats) recipes, 96–102
 Cajun Chicken, 96
 Cheesy Chicken, 97
 Chicken/Beef Mustard, 98
 Chicken Salad, 97
 French Chicken, 98
 Macaroni & Cheese-Tasting Chicken, 99
 Orange-Glazed Duck, 99
 Parmesan Chicken, 100
 Salsa Chicken, 101
 Sexy Chicken, 102
 Tahitian Chicken, 102
 Turkey Pâté, 103
Fowler, Dr. John, 185
freezing of foods, 157
French Chicken (recipe), 98
French Mayonnaise (recipe), 67
French Vanilla Ice Cream (recipe), 131

M

Macaroni & Cheese-Tasting Chicken (recipe), 99
Mango Creamsicles (recipe), 133
marinating raw meats, 50
Mayonnaise (recipes), 67, 71
Meat au Gratin (recipe), 93
meats, raw
    bacteria & parasites in, 19–20
    daily intake of, 39
    defined, 28-30
    in Eskimo diet, 14
    food-combining, 36–37
    function and benefits of, 28–29
    high, 148–149
    marinating, 49
    optimum temperatures for, 27
    preparation of dishes, 61–62
    with raw fats to reverse aging, 21
    recipes (red meat), 87–95
        African Lamb, 88
        Beef Pâté, 89
        Beef Stroganoff, 89
        Carpaccio, 90
        Ethiopian Kitfo, 91
        Himalayan Meat, 87
        Lamb Shanks, 92
        Liver Pâté, 93
        Liver Pâté, Two, 93
        Meat au Gratin, 94
        Nuts Over Meat, 94
        Steak Tartare, 95
    red vs. white
        defined, 29
        different benefits of, 28-29
    sauces for. See sauces for meats
    toxins produced by heating, 152-153
    with unheated honey for digestion, 31
    white meat recipes. See fish/seafood recipes
medicine, allopathic
    deaths and injuries from medications, 8
    modern, 164–165
    origins of, 162–164
    treatments causing disease, 8–9
mercury
    bioactive vs. toxic, 29
    damage caused by, 175

and heavy metals removal (recipe), 56
metabolism
      fast, recommended eating schedule, 41
      slow, recommended eating schedule, 40
metals, heavy (removal formula), 56
Mexican Sour Cream Sauce (recipe), 71
microbes
      as disease eliminators, 170–174
      low levels from drugs & chemicals, 188
microwave packs, 150
milk
      pasteurized, 181–185
      products, optimum temperatures for, 27
      raw
            benefits for infants & children, 181–185
            daily intake of, 39
            food-combining & digestion of, 36
            instead of water, 35
            safety of in scientific studies, 169
            studies supporting health benefits of, 181–183
            as therapeutic treatment, 184–185
Milkshake (recipe), 57
Millstone, Erik, 168
mineral absorption & utilization, 160
Mint Chocolate Substitute (recipe), 127
Moisturizing/Lubrication Drink
      in daily eating program, 40–41
      recipe for, 146
molds, as detoxifying agents, 23
Monroe, Jon, 171
Mornay Sauce (recipe), 72
Morris, Dr. Don, 172
Mousseleine Sauce (recipe), 72
Mushroom Cream Cheese Sauce (recipe), 73
Mushroom Cream Sauce (recipe), 73
mustard, 44
Mustard (recipes), 74–75

N

naps, 24
native diets
      carbohydrates & Native Americans, 31
      Eskimo longevity, 165
      microbes as medicine in, 171–172
      raw fat consumption in, 28
nervous system
      fruit and, 33
      nerve-tissue regeneration, 29

Sweet Cottage Cheese (recipe), 60
Sweet Pickles (recipe), 144
swordfish
mercury and, 29
Swordfish Sashimi (recipe), 112

T

Tahitian Chicken (recipe), 102
Tahitian Fish (recipe), 112
Tango Meat Sauce (recipe), 82
Tartar Coconut Cream Sauce (recipe), 83
Tartar Sauce (recipe), 83
temper, control of, 117
temperature ranges
destruction of nutrients, 153-154
optimum food, 26–27
testes, raw (recipe), 104
Thai Ceviche (recipe), 113
thimerosal, 175
thirst, 35
Thousand Island Meat-Dressing (recipes), 84
Throat Lozenges, Lemon (formula), 147
thyroid gland, raw, 104
Tomato Cream Cheese Sauce (recipe), 85
Tomato Sauce (recipe), 85
tomatoes
food-combining as fruit, 36
with raw fat for dryness and thirst, 35
tooth decay, 21, 169, 182
Toothpaste (formula), 148
toxicity
carcinogens & cooking, 17
as cause of disease, 11–12
removing deep-tissue, 38–43
toxic salts removal (formula), 54
traveling recommendations, 42–43
tuberculosis, pulmonary, 184
tumors, 34, 171, 176
Turkey Pâté (recipe), 103

V

Van Wagtendork, Willem J., 185
Van Winkle, Dr. Elnora, 179
vegetables & vegetable juices. See also juices, green vegetable
acid/alkaline balance and, 151
in cooked diets, 151

PRODUCT-LIST ORDER FORM

Optimal Ways of Living
P.O. Box 176
Santa Monica, CA 90406-0176

Please send me your newest list of producers of raw food products. I enclose a check or money order (not cash) for $15 to cover costs of service, materials and shipping.

(Allow 4-6 weeks for delivery, or much sooner by e-mail.)

Name _____

Address _____

City _____ State _____ Zip _____-_____

Phone #s _____

E-mail Address _____

Your information will not be sold or disclosed to any anyone, including an outside mailing list.

[BOOK ORDER FORM]

USA & Canada TOLL FREE **1-800-247-6553**
International Toll   **1-419-281-1802**

Visa, MasterCard, American Express & Discover Cards accepted

FAX ORDERS
419-281-6883

ON-LINE ORDERS
www.PrimalDiet.com

POSTAL ORDERS
Carnelian Bay Castle Press
c/o BookMasters
P.O. Box 388
Ashland, OH 44805
U.S.A.

Price per book
$29.95*

Sales tax
Ohio residents add 6.25 California residents add 8.25%
SHIPPING
$4.50 for the first book and $2 for each additional book.

Please send: _____ book(s) of The Primal Diet; **We Want To Live.**
Please send: _____ book(s) of **The Recipe For Living Wihtout Disease.**
Name: _____
Address: _____
City: _____ State:_____ Zip:_____

_____ book(s) x $29.95 = _____
(* $39.95 Canada; *Call for International cost and shipping.)
Sales tax   = _____
Shipping: = _____
Total   = _____

Payment   ___ Check ___ Visa   ___ MasterCard
               ___ AMEX   ___ Discover

Card number

_____

Name on card _____ *Exp.date____/____*